The Osteoporotic Syndrome

Detection, Prevention, and Treatment

Fourth Edition

In Memorium

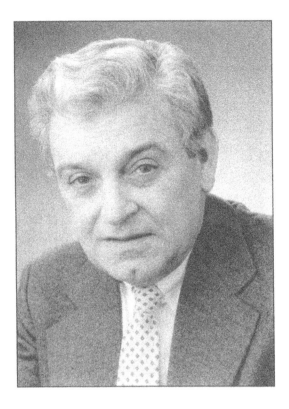

Louis V. Avioli (1931-1999)

Louis V. Avioli, M.D., who conceived and edited the *Osteoporotic Syndrome*, passed away in November, 1999, before this new edition was published. Dr. Avioli was a caring physician and creative scientist with extraordinary energy and a unique ability to communicate. He had a great passion about osteoporosis and he played a critical role in developing and evaluating new approaches to its management. He stimulated public awareness of osteoporosis and was responsible for considerable research that made these new approaches possible. Louis Avioli was a generous and gifted teacher and his many students will continue to have a major influence on the field for decades to come.

Stephen Krane, February, 2000

The Osteoporotic Syndrome

Detection, Prevention, and Treatment

Fourth Edition

EDITED BY

LOUIS V. AVIOLI

Division of Bone and Mineral Diseases
Washington University School of Medicine
St. Louis, Missouri

Academic Press

San Diego   San Francisco   New York   Boston   London   Sydney   Tokyo

Academic Press
A Harcourt Science and Technology Company
525 B Street, Suite 1900, San Diego, California 92101-4495, USA
http://www.apnet.com

Academic Press
24-28 Oval Road, London NW1 7DX, UK
http://www.hbuk.co.uk/ap/

Library of Congress Catalog Card Number: 99-68793

International Standard Book Number: 0-12-068705-4

Printed and bound by CPI Group (UK) Ltd, Croydon, CR0 4YY
Transferred to Digital Print 2011

Contents

Contributors

Numbers in parentheses indicate the pages on which the authors' contributions begin.

Louis V. Avioli
Division of Bone and Mineral Diseases, Washington University School of Medicine, St. Louis, Missouri 63110 (25, 101, 145)

Roberto Civitelli
Division of Bone and Mineral Diseases, Washington University School of Medicine, St. Louis, Missouri 63110 (67)

Bess Dawson-Hughes
Calcium and Bone Metabolism Laboratory, USDA Human Nutrition Research Center, Tufts University, Boston, Massachusetts 02111 (91)

Robert Lindsay
Helen Hayes Hospital, West Haverstraw, New York 10993 (101)

William J. Maloney
Department of Orthopedic Surgery, Washington University School of Medicine, St. Louis, Missouri 63110 (161)

Robert Marcus
Aging Study Unit, Veterans Affairs Medical Center, Stanford University, Palo Alto, California 94304 (173)

Paul D. Miller
Colorado Center for Bone Research, Lakewood, Colorado 80227 (45)

Roberto Pacifici
Division of Bone and Mineral Diseases, Washington University School of Medicine, St. Louis, Missouri 63110 (25)

Linda Repa-Eschen
Division of Bone and Mineral Diseases, Washington University School of Medicine, St. Louis, Missouri 63110 (1)

Clifford J. Rosen
Maine Center for Osteoporosis Research and Education, St. Joseph Hospital, Bangor, Maine 04401 (37)

Stuart L. Silverman
Department of Medicine, University of California at Los Angeles, Beverly Hills, California 90211 (133)

Barbara B. Sterkel
Division of Bone and Mineral Diseases, Washington University School of Medicine, St. Louis, Missouri 63110 (45)

Steven L. Teitelbaum
Division of Bone and Mineral Diseases, Washington University School of Medicine, St. Louis, Missouri 63110 (187)

Nelson B. Watts
Osteoporosis and Bone Health Program, Emory University School of Medicine, Atlanta, Georgia 30322 (121)

Preface

Since the third edition of this volume was published in 1993, considerable knowledge of the ever-escalating magnitude of the osteoporosis problem as a silent disease has been gained. Osteoporosis has become a major health threat, with more than 70 million individuals afflicted in Europe, United States, and Japan alone. With at least 1 in 3 postmenopausal women currently affected by bone loss and/or morbidity caused the osteoporotic syndrome and with health care expenditures in the United States reaching more than $13 billion in 1995, we can anticipate an ever-increasing prevalence of this disorder as the world population increases. The value of early detection and therapeutic intervention with drugs for reversing bone loss has become clear. Because, in the past, fractures and the associated mortality and morbidity were regarded as the most significant clinical manifestations of osteoporosis, it is gratifying that during this time continued study has also established that fracture risk at specific skeletal sites can be assessed easily by noninvasive measurements of bone mineral density. Recognizing the importance of early diagnosis and therapy, the World Health Organization established a quantitative definition of osteoporosis in 1994: a skeletal disorder wherein bone mineral density is more than 2.5 standard deviations below the mean value of normal young adults. Thus, the ability to utilize standardized diagnostic testing not only to identify the patient at risk but also to quantitate the responsive therapy was finally accepted by the medical community as a practical means of approaching the problem of detection and treatment. As illustrated on the cover of this edition, the beneficial effects of estrogen therapy on reversing vertebral structural damage and height loss was demonstrated by Wallach and Henneman forty years ago! Despite these observations, many physicians have ignored preventative estrogen therapy because of a potpourri of concerns that mitigate their enthusiasm for prolonged hormonal intervention. In the 6 years following the publication of the last edition of this volume, a number of new drugs or drug formulations have become available that preserve bone mass and decrease fracture risk without the complications that condition the physicians' use of estrogens for either prevention or therapy of postmenopausal women. These new developments in epidemiology, diagnosis, and treatment have been incorporated into this revised fourth edition of *The Osteoporotic Syndrome*.

Because one of the most significant factors in developing silent osteoporosis is corticosteroid therapy, and because the Medical Bone Mass Measurement Standardization Act of 1998 requires that Medicare pay for bone density testing of patients on corticosteroid therapy, a chapter emphasizing the need for careful monitoring of patients subject to these medications and the appropriate treatment of those hereby destined to lose bone has been added to this edition. Finally, because the nature of the osteoporotic problem often includes orthopedic intervention, the contribution of the orthopedic surgeon to the management of osteoporotic patients is also included in this edition to delineate overall continuity of care.

I extend my thanks and appreciation to the contributors and those individuals who reviewed this edition and provided constructive criticism regarding form and content, to Ms. Judy Pohle for her most capable assistance during the editing and redactory processes, and to the publishers for their limitless patience and understanding.

Louis V. Avioli

1 The Necessity of a Managed Care Approach for Osteoporosis

Linda Repa-Eschen

TAKING CHARGE OF BONE HEALTH

Tuned in, turned on, and taking charge, the female baby boomer, eager to direct care for herself and her family, often accosts her "family doctor" armed with a fistful of "truth" downloaded from the Internet. All too often, the general internist or gynecologist must dispel her fears about breast cancer and the dangers of estrogen while simultaneously balancing contractual gag orders against medical knowledge and the popularized virtues of yams and soy proteins. Pressured by managed care to "practice efficiently," the doc-in-practice hustles through early morning rounds at multiple hospitals—to add more double-booked, appointment-time-slots at the office—where he —or she—scrambles for 10 h between telephone calls and three or four exam rooms—to juggle a panel of "covered lives." For these efforts, he— or she—is phlegmatically informed by a "gray-suit" that an excessive use of "resources" offset the practice's share of the "withhold." The conscientious, albeit harried, physician struggles to balance the acute complications of hypertension, diabetes, heart disease, and cancer with niggling questions about asymptomatic bone loss. An elderly patient's nagging complaints about low back pain is often discounted as an aging woman's reluctance to accept the "normal" consequences of growing old. A middle-aged woman's concerns that she may repeat her mother's history of crippling osteoporosis are often soothed by attributing them to the typical mood swings of "the change" rather than an indicator of her risk for similar bone loss. Osteoporosis is often regarded as a vogue topic for continuing medical education courses with featured "bone" experts. But, this inevitable result of growing old is not a practical priority meriting focused medical evaluation in a hectic private practice. The facts, however, contradict these popular perceptions and will eventually demand a more proactive approach.

QUANTIFYING THE REAL RISK

Nearly 29 million American men and women age 50 and older are currently affected by significant bone loss. These 1997 estimates by the National Osteoporosis Foundation indicate that, for all ethnic groups, more than 10 million Americans already have osteoporosis, and nearly 19 million more have low bone mass and an increased risk for osteoporosis. By 2015 the numbers are expected to swell to more than 41 million Americans either afflicted with or at risk for osteoporosis. However, while bone loss for men and women begins in their thirties, it is not until menopause that bone loss accelerates for women and contributes largely to 1.5 million fractures of the hip, spine, and wrist each year (see Fig. 1-1). Within any given area in the United States, the 29 million affected men and women represent about 13 to 14% of those age 50 and older. Within an individual physician's practice, one in three women who is 50 years of age or older has osteoporosis. Eventually, one out of every two women and one in eight men over the age of 50 will have an osteoporosis-related fracture in his or her lifetime. Surprisingly, in spite of these numbers, only one in four women who is at increased risk for osteoporosis has discussed her bone health with her physician. Osteoporosis is often tagged as a "woman's disease"; there are no studies estimating conversations about osteoporosis between men and their physicians.

Data from the National Health, Nutrition, and Educational Survey III (NHANES III) have been used to extrapolate estimates of prevalence of bone loss among various ethnic groups (see Table 1-1) and can serve as indicators of local prevalence rates in a given locale. Estimating the prevalence rates among men is more difficult, and ranges vary from between a high of 24%

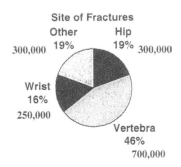

Fig. 1-1. Percentage distribution of the 1.5 million annual osteoporotic fractures in the United States. Source: Data adapted from National Osteoporosis Foundation, 1998.

TABLE 1-1. Percentage of Women Age 50 and Older by Ethnic Group

Ethnic Group	Low Bone Mineral Density(%)	Osteoporosis (%)
Non-Hispanic White and Asian	39	21
American Indian and Hispanic	36	16
Black	29	10

Source: Data adapted from "1996 and 2015 Osteoporosis Prevalence Figures, State-by-State Report," National Osteoporosis Foundation, January 1997.

for white men 80 years of age and older to a low of 5% for men of similar age from Asian, Hispanic, and American Indian heritage. More specifically, while there are wide geographical variations in the incidence of hip fractures worldwide, they are higher among white women living in northern Europe, particularly Sweden, and North America, including the United States, than in Asian or black populations. Overall, 1996 prevalence figures for all ethnic groups of those 50 and older indicate that of the 29 million affected Americans, 23.5 million women and 5.2 million men have either low bone mass or established osteoporosis. Some osteoporosis experts have estimated even greater prevalence among white, postmenopausal women alone, with as many as 9.4 million having osteoporosis and 16.8 million having osteopenia, that is, a vertebral bone mineral density (BMD) value in women below -1.0 to -2.49 standard deviations. Marketing studies from the pharmaceutical industry estimate that as many as 21 million Americans have established osteoporosis, that is, a vertebral BMD value less than -2.50 standard deviations. Consensus among all estimates, though, projects that as few as 20% have been diagnosed and as few as 5%—or a little over 1 million—are actually receiving treatment.

A targeted screening program aimed at those women 50 and older could identify many of the undiagnosed 80%, or more than 16 million Americans. Comparatively, of the 50 million Americans with hypertension, almost two out of three have been diagnosed, and as many as one-half are being treated. *In contrast, 9 of the 10 individuals—or 20 million Americans—with significant bone loss currently receive no treatment.* In its early, asymptomatic stages, osteoporosis is not a sexy disease: its complications are uneventful and demand minimal medical intervention—hardly meriting the focused attention of well-honed medical acumen or the focused intervention of physicians harried by the demands of practice. Too often, the pain of an acute fracture prompts the diagnosis of osteoporosis. At this point, the targeted outcome of treatment is to stabilize the patient, prevent additional bone loss and new fractures, and attempt to strengthen an already debilitated skeleton.

The "approved" medical model for managing osteoporosis emphasizes symptomatic disease, acute "fracture" events, and vertebral bone loss so excessive as to be at least -2.5 standard deviations below the average for a young person of comparable age. Unfortunately, many third party payers have restricted their litmus test for payment related to bone loss and the management of bone health to this narrow definition and quantifiable measure of osteoporosis: any bone density value between 1 and 2.5 standard deviations below the reference group mean for a young normal (T-score) is defined as "osteopenia"—a diagnosis of early bone loss for which the measurement of bone mineral density is considered by most third party payers to be medically "unnecessary" and therefore "uncovered." This pervasive "standard of care" for osteoporosis identifies only one out of every five individuals as having the disease and targets treatment for only five of every 100 afflicted. This practice is comparable to sticking an occasional Band-Aid on a truckload of cracked eggs, with the amount of eggs expected to multiply exponentially in the next 50 years.

GROWING NUMBERS MAGNIFY THE PROBLEM

In 1999, about 27% or 72 million of the U.S. population was over the age of 50, with those 65 and older comprising about 13% or nearly one in every eight Americans. By 2001 there will be over 80 million Americans over the age of 50 who will consume about 70% percent of the health care resources. Every 8 sec another of the 77 million baby boomers turns 50. By 2010, when the baby boomers begin to turn 65, "older" Americans will represent 20% or one in five of the population. As this wave of individuals born between 1946 and 1964 ages, the elderly population is likely to double by 2030. Similarly, minority populations, often inaccurately regarded as immune from significant bone loss, are projected to make up 25% of the elderly population. On average, women live 7 years longer than men and currently represent 59% of those over age 65 and 71% of those 85 and older. Today, the average Medicare patient "manages" three to four chronic conditions. Tomorrow, as their longevity increases and as a larger percentage of the population is 65 and older, the drain on limited health care resources to manage their chronic conditions will swell. Gradually, the advances of medical science are transforming the practice of medicine away from treatment for acute, isolated incidents to a series of encounters for the management of chronic diseases (see Fig. 1-2). Without targeted, interventive strategies, one of those chronic conditions will certainly be osteoporosis.

DEFINING COST

In 1995 estimates of the direct costs for osteoporotic fractures topped nearly $14 billion per annum and included inpatient hospitalization, nursing home care, and outpatient care. These estimates indicate that osteoporosis-related fractures accounted for about 4% of all Medicare costs with two-thirds of the costs resulting from hip fractures. Currently only 9.4% of the

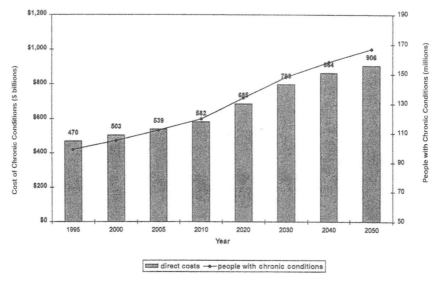

Fig. 1-2. Predicted increase in prevalence and cost of chronic conditions in the United States, from 1995 to 2050. Source: Data adapted from National Center for Health Statistics, 1995.

costs related to osteoporosis are for outpatient care, with preventive intervention nearly nonexistent (see Fig. 1-3). While the gradual loss of bone occurs much earlier than the seventh decade, its acute effects and their economic impact in the United States are borne primarily by the elderly, Medicare, and, increasingly, privately owned Medicare risk providers. Eighty-eight percent of the costs associated with osteoporosis are for patients 65 years of

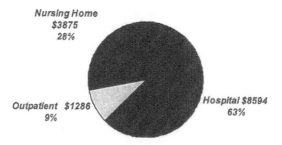

Fig. 1-3. Health care expenditures ($millions) for osteoporotic fractures in the Unites States by type of service. Total estimated expenditures for 1995 were $13.764 billion. Source: Data adapted from Melton LJ, *et al.*: Medical expenditures for the treatment of osteoporotic fractures in the United States in 1995: Report from the National Osteoporosis Foundation. J Bone Miner Res 12:24–37, 1997.

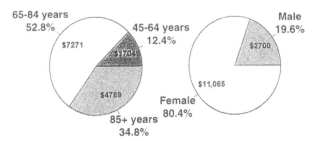

Fig. 1-4. Health care expenditures ($millions) for osteoporotic fractures in the Unites States by sex and age distribution. Total estimated expenditures for 1995 were $13.764 billion. Source: Data adapted from Melton LJ, *et al.*: Medical expenditures for the treatment of osteoporotic fractures in the United States in 1995: Report from the National Osteoporosis Foundation. J Bone Miner Res 12:24–37, 1997.

age and older (see Fig. 1-4). If this trend continues, the annual cost of osteoporosis may be as much as $62 billion by the year 2020. While those 85 and older comprise only 11% of nondisabled Medicare enrollees, they use a much larger relative portion of the resources, accounting for nearly $4.8 billion or 35% of the estimated $14 billion (see Fig. 1-4). Demographically, women make up 59% of the Medicare enrollees and over 70% of those 85 and older (see Fig. 1-5). Relatedly, women account for 84% of the $4.8 billion expended on osteoporotic fractures in that age group.

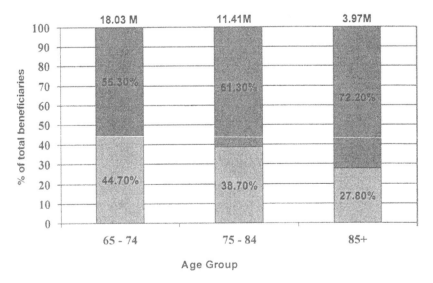

Fig. 1-5. Medicare beneficiaries by age and sex. Light shading, male; dark shading, female. Source: Data adapted from Health Care Financing Administration, 1997.

Studies estimate that the probability that a woman alive at age 50 years will be hospitalized with a hip fracture at least once before she dies, is 11.6%. Estimates of the lifetime risk are 15 to 16%. Some estimate that 54% of 50-year-old women will experience an osteoporosis-related fracture during their remaining years. Those over 65 account for the majority of the 300,000 annual hip fractures in the United States and the 1.7 million worldwide. In 1992–1994, three out of five injury-related hospitalizations for elderly persons 75 and older were for fracture with more than one-half of those being hip fractures. On discharge, 17 to 52% of hip fracture patients are sent to a nursing home. As many as one-third of those admitted to nursing homes for temporary stays remained institutionalized 1 year later, and one in five hip fracture patients will die within the first 6 months after the fracture incident. Estimates of the percentage of these patients with hip fractures who regain their former level of health range from 22 to 83%. In fact, only half of these individuals will regain their ability to walk independently for as short a distance as 20 feet. Disability following hip fracture is even higher worldwide, with as many as two-thirds of Asian victims remaining disabled after 1 year of the fracture. Although there are significant geographical differences in the incidence of hip fracture worldwide, hip fractures increase proportionately as socioeconomic levels rise and longevity increases.

Of the estimated $14 billion spent on osteoporotic fractures, fully $8.7 billion or nearly two-thirds results from hip fractures. For the individual patient the estimated cost of a hip fracture ranges from $30,850 to $33,428. From a cost-for-treatment perspective alone, were this money to be spent on the early detection and treatment of low bone density rather than on the consequences of end-stage disease, this same patient and three friends could theoretically at age 55 be treated for 21 years, until the age of 76, with hormone replacements, or for about 11 years with either alendronate or raloxifene. A small reduction in the incidence of hip fractures in treated individuals could save thousands of lives and several millions of dollars each year.

MANAGING BONE HEALTH IN A MANAGED CARE ENVIRONMENT

In a health care environment dominated by managed care, the ever escalating costs of caring for patients with chronic illnesses demand a medically proactive and financially prudent strategy of management. For osteoporosis, a cost-effective strategy promotes "wellness" by emphasizing attainment of peak bone mineral density, identifying risk, detecting low bone mass in a quality-controlled environment, managing advanced disease, and educating physicians and patients. Targeting the "bone health" needs of women at early postmenopause can provide a cost-effective way to intervene before the appearance of fracture symptoms at the end stage of disease later in life. As managed care dominates the delivery of health care, prevention becomes the only strategy for managing the complications of advanced disease by lengthening the period of active life expectancy, reducing fractures, and minimizing the costs resulting from hip fractures. In its early stages of development, managed care in this country could easily control costs by restricting enrollment to the healthy, limiting the number of hospitalizations, reducing length of stay, consolidating delivery systems, and controlling units of service by reviewing clinical processes. However, as managed care penetration nears 70 or 80% of the population in a given area, the health risks of the panel of insured lives will reflect those public health problems of the larger population. The key to continued physical and financial viability for the population and both private and Medicare HMOs will be early identification of those at high risk for particular diseases, particularly osteoporosis, as some form of managed care will continue to dominate the delivery of care in this country.

Targeting Costs by Identifying Risk— Availability of Bone Mass Measurements

An essential and cost-effective care plan to identify low bone mass in men and women must include targeted measurements of bone mineral density (BMD). Bone mass measurements remain the most accurate predictor of fracture risk, with BMD measurements at the hip, rather than at other skeletal sites, being the most accurate for predicting hip fracture. Prior to July 1998, 96% of Medicare carriers routinely denied claims for bone mass measurements, particularly if submitted with the diagnoses "osteopenia," "compression fractures of the vertebrae," or "drug-induced osteoporosis." Coverage for the conditions that most negatively affect bone were routinely denied. Only 4% of Medicare carriers approved claims for "postmenopausal estrogen deficiency," and only 20% approved "vertebral X-ray abnormalities" or "pathologic fractures."

As of July 1, 1998, Medicare effectively standardized its policies regulating its standards for reimbursement for measurements of bone mineral density among all of its 58 regional carriers. According to the ruling of the Health Care Financing Administration (HCFA), "bone mass measurements, using bone densitometers and bone sonometers, are considered to be the most valuable objective indicator of the risk of fracture and/or osteoporosis. The clinical use of these devices is based on the assumption that bone mass is an important determinant of osteoporotic fractures, and that bone mass measurements may help reduce the number of fractures by identifying high-risk individuals, who can then receive appropriate preventive measures. Because osteoporosis is generally considered preventable, but not reversible . . . early detection of at-risk individuals is a desirable health outcome" (*Federal Register,* 06/24/98, p. 34320).

The expansion of Medicare coverage to include preventative benefits for bone mass measurements is a clear indicator of Congressional intent to improve the overall health of "qualified" individuals and reduce the escalating costs of Medicare. Tables 1-2 and 1-3 itemize the medical indications

**TABLE 1-2. Billing Codes and Reimbursement Rates
for Bone Density Technologies**

cpt Code	Procedure	Site	Fee Schedule Amount[a]
76075	DEXA (*dual-energy X-ray absorptiometry*)	Axial	$131.35
76076	pDEXA (*peripheral DXA*)	Appendicular	$40.72
76078	RA (*radiographic absorptiometry*)	Appendicular	$39.99
78350	SPA (*single photon absorptiometry*)	Appendicular	$40.72
G0130	SXA (*single-energy X-ray absorptiometry*)	Appendicular	$40.72
G0131	QCT (*quantitative computed tomography*)	Axial	$124.00
G0132	pQCT (*peripheral QCT*)	Appendicular	$40.72
G0133	QUS (*quantitative ultrasound*)	Appendicular	$40.72

[a]National average, effective July 1, 1998; subject to local variations and periodic updates.

(Table 1-3) for BMDs to link with the respective cpt (common procedural terminology) (Table 1-2) codes. At the time of the claims' submission, payment is contingent on accurately linking the diagnosis code for the medical indication with the appropriate cpt code as noted in Table 1-3. Inconsistent practices of denying claims for measurements of bone mineral density permeate commercial insurance companies and managed care plans. The "lack of medical necessity" is the most frequently cited reason for denial although some insurance carriers still refuse payment on the charge that BMDs are "experimental procedures." Because the approved cpt codes have changed three times since July of 1996, many carriers have lagged behind in updating their databases for approved codes resulting in even more confusion and denials for payment due to "inaccurate coding."

National Medicare reimbursement rates for the various approved technologies and their respective cpt codes are noted in Table 1-2. Although the HCFA projects that the effect of this rule will result in expenditures of greater than $100 million beginning in fiscal year 1999, the net effects of this new rule on Medicare beneficiaries will be very positive. Through earlier detection of low bone mass and the use of appropriate prevention and treatment measures, the HCFA projects an eventual reduction in the ravaging effects of osteoporosis among the Medicare population. In providing for this broad-based preventive benefit, Medicare has restricted the frequency of BMD measurements to once every 24 months for all individuals covered by Medicare plans, including Medicare risk contracts with managed care corporations. With substantiation of medical necessity, reimbursement for follow-up measurements of BMD to follow response to therapy may also be approved.

Practice Patterns Using Bone Mineral Densities

Because of its precision, diagnostic accuracy, and the widespread availability of dual-energy X-ray absorptiometry (DEXA) equipment throughout

TABLE 1-3. Commonly Used Diagnoses for Bone Loss[a]

Diagnosis Codes	Primary Diagnosis
252.0	Hyperparathyroidism
256.2	Postablative ovarian failure
256.3	Other ovarian failure (premature menopause NOS, primary ovarian failure
259.3	Ectopic hormone secretion, not elsewhere classified (hyperparathyroidism)
268.2	Osteomalacia, unspecified
275.3	Disorders of phosphorus metabolism (osteomalacia, hypophophatasia)
626.0	Absence of menstruation (amenorrhea)
627.0–627.8	Menopausal and postmenopausal disorders
627.0	Premenopausal menorrhagia
627.1	Postmenopausal bleeding
627.2	Menopausal or female climacteric states
627.3	Postmenopausal atrophic vaginitis
627.4	States associated with artificial menopause
627.8	Other specified menopausal and postmenopausal disorders (excludes 256.3)
733.0	Osteoporosis, unspecified
733.01	Senile osteoporosis
733.02	Idiopathic osteoporosis
733.09	Osteoporosis, other (drug-induced)
733.13	Pathologic fracture of vertebrae
733.90	Osteopenia
805.20	Fracture of thoracic spine, closed
806.40	Fracture of lumbar spine, closed
V56.69	Encounter for long-term (current) use of other medications (prednisone > 7.5 or less per day for 3 months) (monitoring to assess response, efficacy of an FDA-approved osteoporosis drug therapy).

[a] Check with your regional Medicare carrier to identify those ICD-9 CM codes that support medical necessity. Those listed here are from the Missouri General American Life Insurance Company, the administrator of the Medicare program for the northeast portion of Missouri. Policy revision number 8, start date of notice 09/25/98. Bone Density Measurement Policy Identifier, no. 47, p. 4. See ICD-9 CM 9th revision, Clinical Modification, 5th edition. Los Angeles: PMIC, 1999.

U.S. metropolitan areas, DEXA is the most widely used procedure for diagnosing patients with suspected disease or clinical symptoms and for guiding decisions about treatment. In 1997 the HCFA received 781,593 Medicare claims for measurements of BMD, with 93% (727,561) of those for axial measurements of the hip or spine. Measurements of BMD, of the appendicular or peripheral skeleton made up only 7% of all Medicare claims. Sixty-nine percent (539,811) were submitted as "global" charges that included both technical and professional components (see Table 1-4). Internal medicine

TABLE 1-4. Number of Claims for Payment Submitted in 1997 to Medicare for Measurements of Bone Mineral Density by Skeletal Site and Type of Service Using CPT Codes 76075, 76076, and Modifiers TC and 26[a]

Type of Service	Skeletal Site				Grand Total	
	Axial	%	Peripheral	%	Total Number	%
Global	511,017	65.39	28,794	3.68	539,811	69.07
Technical component only	24,544	3.14	3722	0.48	28,266	3.62
Professional component only	191,879	24.55	21,456	2.75	213,335	27.30
Other	121	0.02	0	0.00	121	0.02
Grand total	727,561 (93.09%)	68.53	53,972 (6.9096%)	6.91	781,533	100.00

Source: Health Care Financing Administration, at www.hcfa.gov (12/9/98), Statistics & Data, "1999 Resource Based Practice Expense Data Files."
[a] Measurements of bone mineral density consist of two separate services and result in two distinct charges: (1) a technical component, which refers to the performance of the procedure itself and is usually performed by a radiologic technologist (RT); and (2) a professional component, which refers to the radiological supervision and interpretation of the procedure and is performed by the attending physician. If these components are billed together as one fee, the claim is referred to as "global." The claim is submitted with the appropriate cpt code or 76075 or 76076; there are no modifiers. If the claim is submitted as two distinct charges, the technical portion is submitted with the modifier "TC" after the cpt code, as 76075-TC; the professional portion is submitted with the modifier "26" after the cpt code, as 76075-26.

specialists are the predominant providers of BMDs, having submitted nearly 57% (306,711) of all global claims and 45% (351,742) of all individual technical or professional claims (Table 1-5). See Tables 1-6 and 1-7 for an itemized listing of providers of BMDs by medical specialty. Market survey data of 1565 providers indicate that internal medicine and women's health specialists are the predominant providers for BMD measurements (see Figs. 1-6, 1-7, and 1-8,) as they integrate clinical management of the patient with technical supervision of the technique. Both survey and Medicare claims data suggest that the predominant practice is for bone health specialists who evaluate and manage the patient also to interpret and supervise the technical efficacy of the BMD measurements. Ensuring the technical efficacy of BMD measurements requires accurate, precise, and reproducible results between various equipment and among different operators. Wide discrepancy between the values obtained from different BMD measurement units at different centers demonstrate variability of as much as 3.5 standard deviations in results. The varying precision among operators often results in widely divergent results. Patients diagnosed with severe osteoporosis (exceeding -3.5 standard deviations below the mean for an age-matched normal) using one DEXA device are often determined to be normal using quality-controlled procedures.

TABLE 1-5. Number of Global Claims Submitted in 1997 to Medicare by Specialty for Measurements of Bone Mineral Density Using CPT Codes 76075 and 76076, Axial and Peripheral Skeletal Sites

Specialty	Frequency	
	Number	%
Internal medicine	306,711	56.82
General/family practice	6729	1.247
Clinics/groups	21,194	3.926
Neurology	237	0.044
Otolaryngology	210	0.039
Pediatrics	30	0.006
Physical medicine	2131	0.395
Subtotal—medicine related specialties	30,531	5.66
Radiology	117,728	21.809
Obstetrics/gynecology	21,930	4.063
Surgery	28,796	5.334
Independent physicians' lab	167	0.031
All others	33,948	6.289
Grand total	539,811	100.00

Source: Health Care Financing Administration, at www.hcfa.gov (12/9/98) Statistics & Data, "1999 Resource Based Practice Expense Data Files."

Managing Health Care Delivery

The implementation of Medicare's coverage for bone mass measurements endorses the widespread belief, at least in the United States, that early detection and management of disease can lead to substantial reductions in life-threatening and serious illness and in the escalating financial costs of hip fractures. By targeting high-risk individuals for appropriate intervention, the federal government is taking a leading role in managing the risks for osteoporosis. Similarly, as market penetration of managed care approaches 70 to 80% of the insured population, managed care corporations will be forced to adopt "best practice" care plans that can succeed in identifying and managing health care risks before the onset of advanced disease, fractures, and the markedly added costs of treatment.

Managing Cost While Managing Risk—Medicare Risk Contracts

In its attempts to manage these costs, the HCFA has also expanded its financial incentives to private industry to encourage its participation in Medicare by offering to pay 95% of the approved fee schedule, regardless of utilization, for managing the care of its Medicare enrollees. In 1990 only 8% of the more than 60 million Medicare and Medicaid recipients were enrolled in Medicare HMOs. Eight years later in December of 1998, more than 18% or

TABLE 1-6. Number of Claims Submitted in 1997 to Medicare by Medical Specialty for Measurements of Bone Mineral Density Using CPT Codes 76075, 76076, and Modifiers TC and 26, Axial and Peripheral Skeletal Sites[a]

Specialty	Frequency		
	Number	%	Cumulative %
Internal medicine	351,742	45.01	45.01
General/family practice	34,950	4.472	49.48
Clinics/groups	34,422	4.404	53.88
Neurology	1000	0.128	54.01
Otolaryngology	300	0.038	54.05
Pediatrics	466	0.060	54.11
Physical medicine	2223	0.284	54.39
Subtotal—medicine related specialties	73,361	9.39	
Radiology	278,806	35.67	90.07
Obstetrics/gynecology	23,453	3.00	93.07
Surgery	31,729	4.06	97.13
Independent physician's lab	17.323	2.22	99.35
All others	5119	0.65	100.00
Grand total	781,533	100.00	

Source: Health Care Financing Administration, at www.hcfa.gov (12/9/98) Statistics & Data, "1999 Resource Based Practice Expense Data Files."
[a]Measurements of bone mineral density consist of two separate services and result in two distinct charges: (1) a technical component, which refers to the performance of the procedure itself and is usually performed by a radiologic technologist (RT); and (2) a professional component, which refers to the radiological supervision and interpretation of the procedure and is performed by the attending physician. If these components are billed together as one fee, the claim is referred to as "global." The claim is submitted with the appropriate cpt code or 76075 or 76076; there are no modifiers. If the claim is submitted as two distinct charges, the technical portion is submitted with the modifier "TC" after the cpt code, as 76075-TC; the professional portion is submitted with the modifier "26" after the cpt code, as 76075-26.

6.7 million of Medicare recipients were enrolled in risk contracts, with the number of contracts since 1990 nearly tripling (see Fig. 1-9). In April 1998 alone more than 100,000 beneficiaries enrolled in Medicare HMOs. Estimates for 1998 indicated that every 30 sec, one senior joins an HMO—seeking lower costs and more benefits. With the dramatic increase of Medicare risk HMO plans being offered by the dominant companies, such as Aetna/USHC, United HealthCare, and BCBS Plans, the "trickle-down" mimicry of Medicare's benefits by privately owned insurance companies may speed more widespread availability of coverage of measurements of BMD. As managed care struggles to maintain shrinking margins while insuring a representative population of enrollees, it is becoming strikingly obvious that providing cost-effective preventive benefits is more financially prudent than treating advanced disease.

TABLE 1-7. Number of Claims Submitted in 1997 to Medicare by Medical Subspecialty for Measurements of Bone Mineral Density Using CPT Codes 76075, 76076, and Modifiers TC and 26

Specialty	Frequency		
	Number	%	Cumulative %
General internal medicine	145,234	18.583	18.583
Allergy/immunology	2149	0.275	18.858
Cardiology	3669	0.469	19.328
Dermatology	142	0.018	19.346
Gastroenterology	1365	0.175	19.520
Pulmonary	4655	0.596	20.116
Geriatrics	894	0.114	20.230
Nephrology	5928	0.759	20.989
Infectious diseases	949	0.121	21.110
Endocrinology	51,696	6.615	27.725
Rheumatology	133,166	17.039	44.764
Hematology	32	0.004	44.768
Hematology/oncology	955	0.122	44.890
Preventive medicine	10	0.001	44.892
Medical oncology	298	0.038	44.930
Emergency medicine	600	0.077	45.007
Subtotal internal medicine	351,742	45.007	
General family practice	34,950	4.472	49.479
Clinics/groups	34,422	4.404	53.883
Neurology	1000	0.128	54.011
Otolaryngology	300	0.038	54.049
Pediatrics	466	0.060	45.109
Physical medicine	2223	0.284	54.393
Radiology	247,826	31.710	86.104
Nuclear medicine	25,790	3.300	89.404
Mammography	14	0.002	89.405
Independent lab	182	0.023	89.429
Radiation oncology	54	0.007	89.436
Interventional radiology	4940	0.632	90.068
Subtotal radiology	278,806	35.674	
Obstetrics/gynecology	23,453	3.001	93.07
Surgery—general surgery	1085	0.139	93.207
Orthopedic surgery	30,267	3.873	97.080
Thoracic surgery	275	0.035	97.115
Hand surgery	76	0.010	97.125
Urology	26	0.003	97.128
Subtotal—surgery	31,729	4.060	
Independent physicians' lab	17,323	2.217	99.345
All others	5119	0.655	100.00
Grand total	781,533	100.00	100.00

Source: Health Care Financing Administration, at www.hcfa.gov (12/9/98) Statistics & Data, "1999 Resource Based Practice Expense Data Files."

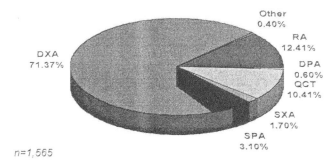

Fig. 1-6. Percentage distribution of BMD scanner types in U.S. centers. Source: Data derived from Merck Pharmaceuticals, 1996, Market Survey of U.S. BMD Scanners.

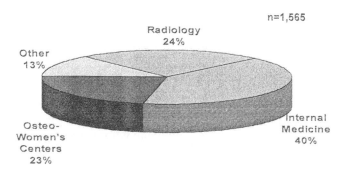

Fig. 1-7. Percentage distribution of BMD scanner location by specialty. Source: Data derived from Merck Pharmaceuticals, 1996, Market Survey of U.S. BMD Scanners.

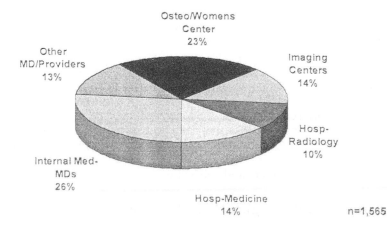

Fig. 1-8. Percentage distribution of BMD scanner location by providers. Source: Data derived from Merck Pharmaceuticals, 1996, Market Survey of U.S. BMD Scanners.

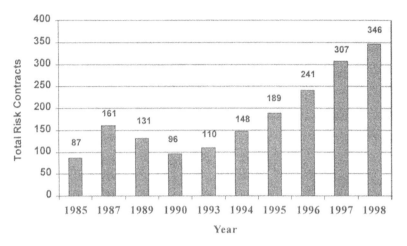

Fig. 1-9. Medicare risk contracts from 1985 to 1997. Source: Health Care Financing Administration. Note that not all years are included.

Managing Risks Rather Than Managing Disease

A promising avenue for substantial reduction in costs depends on preventing bone loss and its subsequent fractures rather than on improving the treatment of patients with fractures. A woman whose hip bone density is one standard deviation below the mean for her age is about seven times more likely to have a hip fracture than a woman whose bone density is one standard deviation above the mean. Administrators, physicians, and third-party payers must begin to acknowledge the fact that the impact of osteoporosis on health care costs is sufficient to justify prevention *if a suitable program can be defined!* The ideal program would focus on wellness by integrating "bone health" services throughout the life span to reduce and manage risk and thereby improve health and functional mobility. The components of a comprehensive program may include (1) a cost-effective screening plan; (2) accurate and precise methods for quantifying bone mineral density for the detection of early bone loss and for monitoring response to therapy; (3) early identification of the risk factors which condition bone loss and fractures; (4) early identification of those individuals who are at greatest risk for osteoporosis; (5) prescription of targeted intervention, as needed; (6) utilization of treatments for osteoporosis that have been approved by the appropriate health care officials; (7) education of physicians and the public to increase knowledge and mobilize response; and (8) integrated referral systems between primary care providers and specialists.

Managing Risk Strategically at Menopause

With either surgical or "natural" menopause (mean age 51 years), bone loss accelerates greatly, with as much as 20% of a woman's bone mass being silently lost within 5 to 7 years following menopause. With the widespread availability of precise and accurate methods to quantitate bone mineral density, this natural event of aging has been shown to occur much earlier than expected. In 1971, the first National Health, Nutrition, and Educational Survey (NHANES I) reported observations of decreased bone mass of the middle phalanx of the little finger in 6 to 18% of women between the ages of 25 and 34. More recent studies substantiate that for some women vertebral bone loss begins before menses cease, especially in those women with altered menstrual function. Evidence is clear that silent and progressive bone loss occurs gradually—as we age—and not suddenly, when we are labeled "elderly" at 65, the dawn of retirement and Medicare eligibility. In this regard it should be noted that although rates of bone loss in women exceed those of men between 50 and 65, after age 65, men and women tend to lose bone at about the same rate. By strategically targeting an effective screening program at identifying the risk for osteoporosis during the perimenopause or with identification of significant risk factors, appropriate intervention can effectively eliminate disease. Authorization and payment for quantifying "low bone mass" with BMD measurements is often, though, denied by non-Medicare carriers as being "medically unnecessary" in both men and perimenopausal women.

Targeted Screening

Currently, claims for tests and procedures to "rule out" or to "screen" for disease are regarded as costly and inconclusive, and they are routinely denied. "Screening" is often inaccurately defined by those who refuse to acknowledge the impact of the osteoporosis problem as "mass" testing of an entire population. In fact, cost-effectively implemented, screening is the systematic examination of *selected* patients *at risk for* disease in order to determine their suitability for either initiating intervention or continuing treatment. Peak bone density and rate of bone loss are important determinants of individual bone density in advanced age. Studies have demonstrated that a woman at age 50 with bone density measurements of the hip in the tenth percentile, as measured by dual energy radiography (DEXA), has a 25% lifetime risk for a hip fracture. A decrease of one standard deviation in bone mass is associated with a 50–100% increase in fracture incidence. On the other hand, if that same 50-year-old woman measures in the ninetieth percentile, her risk for a hip fracture is reduced to 6%—a 4.3-fold reduction in her relative risk for a hip fracture.

While perimenopausal screening with BMD would likely result in greater numbers of women being treated for a longer periods of time than if assessments began at age 65, its cost-effectiveness is questionable, prompting many experts to limit screening to elderly populations. However, one study has estimated the cost of testing 50 million adults annually with BMD to be $3.75 billion. Thus, when compared to the previously quoted $8.7 billion spent annually on hip fractures, the development of a targeted screening program for high-risk individuals could result in substantial savings. Focusing on high-risk, early postmenopausal women, a pilot program might include a three-step process: (1) use of a simple, prescreening questionnaire to identify key risk factors as indicators for follow-up; (2) use of appendicular bone density measurements—possibly with an ultrasound sonometer of the calcaneus—as a broad-based screening tool; and, if indicated, (3) a central DEXA of the hip and spine followed by targeted intervention and/or treatment for those with low BMD or established osteoporosis. Structuring the use of assessment tools and procedures in progressive, decisional tiers enables physicians to make informed judgments based on the results of previous tests and the differential diagnosis of the accumulated data.

Developing Referral Systems and Coordinated Care Plans between the Primary Care Provider and Specialist

With the widespread availability of DEXA and increased managed care penetration, the role of the bone health specialist is more narrowly defined and usually includes measurement of bone mineral density and evaluation and management consultation. While the primary care provider (PCP) is key to identifying the patient at high risk of developing osteoporosis, studies indicate that the use of bone mineral densitometry by most physicians is low. In fact, one study showed that 38% of PCPs and 32% of gynecologists never used BMD measurements in early postmenopausal women. The most important criteria for those PCPs and gynecologists who do use BMD measurements are the presence of risk factors which they associate with chronic glucocorticoid use and recent fractures. By partnering with the PCP and managed care plans, the specialist can develop "best practice" plans for managing bone health throughout life. Many patients referred to specialists present with advanced bone disease and multiple diagnoses requiring coordinated and detailed care plans and the continued medical management of a PCP. While the primary presenting diagnosis is "osteoporosis," the management plan is often complicated by a history of carcinoma or organ transplant necessitating ongoing management with "bone wasting" drugs. A recent study indicates that clinical reporting which includes interpretation of the BMD and a care plan, rather than brief technical reports of BMD results, increased the PCP's use and understanding of bone densitometry and actually changed the PCP's management of the patient.

Managing Education

For integrated health systems to be cost effective, it is essential to expand the role of the consumer in managing disease and the role of the physician in educating patients. Evidence indicates that patient education is essential both for prevention and for assuring compliance with treatment which may extend for many years. One study showed that a bone mineral density test, regardless of the result, had a significant effect on women's decisions to accept hormone replacement therapy (HRT), and that women with lower BMD were more likely to choose HRT. A number of studies show that patients' compliance with medical management is highly correlated with the frequency and effectiveness of personal education by the physician. The acceptance of HRT by skeptical women has been shown to be strongly related to interactions with their physicians. Yet, according to a Gallup poll, 75% of women ages 45 to 75 have never talked with a doctor about osteoporosis— even if they were later found to be at significantly greater risk for early bone loss. Targeted education can influence actions regarding health care and decisions about treatment. By partnering together, health care systems, PCPs, and specialists should devise both practice- and community-based educational programs for intervention at key developmental stages in bone health rather than restricting interventions to symptomatic, end-stage disease.

Managing the Care of an Elderly Osteoporotic Population

Because of the distinctive characteristics and special needs of the elderly, it is important to recognize age-related differences in the delivery of health care services which increase the frequency and utilization of resources for this population. Nearly one-half of the patient population of a typical bone health program is 65 years of age and older. Because the "treatment" of osteoporosis has focused on visually identifiable stages of advanced disease, the typical age of a patient referred with osteoporosis to the bone health diagnostic service is postmenopausal and elderly. The difficulties of delivering appropriate care for the elderly is often confounded by multiple chronic conditions and related drug regimens. Sensory impairment, including visual impairment, hearing loss, and incontinence, confound the problem and demand specialized training for both medical support and clerical staffs. Since communication and comprehension are often difficult, interactions between patients, primary care physicians, and bone health consultants often require a lengthy history and physical examination and a coordinated triage. Because of the presence of coexisting diseases, therapeutic intervention for osteoporosis must be carefully monitored and coordinated with the PCP. Compliance is difficult since administration of therapy for the osteoporotic problem must be coordinated with the use of other drug regimens. Controlling disease, monitoring effectiveness of multiple therapeutic regimens, preventing adverse polypharmaceutical interactions, maintaining independence and autonomy with supportive education, and insuring an active lifestyle may require more frequent office visits to a broader variety of health care professionals. Managing chronic disease is not a single, acute event that occurs in a given point in time. It is an ongoing process of health care interventions extended over time. By implementing patient education programs, such as support groups, Internet chat rooms, and targeted newsletters, it may be possible to enable patients themselves to live healthier lives by actively engaging the patient in the management of his or her health. By partnering with community-based organizations and health care systems, health care providers may integrate standards of "best practices" throughout the spectrum of health services.

Managed Care Can Be Managing Care

For most physicians, their medical school and postdoctoral education has primarily focused on the patient as presenting with acute problems, such as a fracture, requiring specialized treatments or targeted intervention. Similarly, the financing of health care had traditionally been structured as fees-for-services for particular acute events and their related consequences. Gradually, the financing for health care has shifted to fixed payment models and capitated fees for the management of "covered lives," so that a typical health care encounter has been shifting from treatment for an acute incident to a series of encounters for the management of chronic diseases. Theoretically, for chronically ill patients with established osteoporosis, the best care is "managed" care which can implement "best practice" plans for coordinated care across multiple medical disciplines and diverse spectrums of a chronic disease process. If managed care, though, is merely managing costs by channeling patients to the cheapest provider, then patient care is often viewed as isolated incidents of care. Access and utilization are, then, often denied. If the focus is simply on cost controls, then, the chronically ill patient is often underserved or ignored.

CONCLUSION

Since 1990 large HMOs, with 200,000 or more members, continue to capture the majority of enrollees (see Fig. 1-10). With the continued consolidation of managed care offerings within a relatively small number of carriers, widespread implementation of strategies to target prevention of major public health problems, such as osteoporosis, is both savvy economics and sound public health policy. The once open-ended benefits in traditional fee-for-service models have over the years been largely replaced with defined benefits based on set contributions. By the end of 1998, more than 61% of insured Americans receive medical care through some form of managed care. More than 85% of working Americans were enrolled in some type of managed care plan. For the elderly, nearly 18% were covered by Medicare HMOs. In all sectors the movement has been to shift cost and responsibility to the individual provider and patient. The best approach is a fully integrated, systems model which targets improvement of health and positive outcomes. Cost-effective care is patient-focused through multidisciplinary

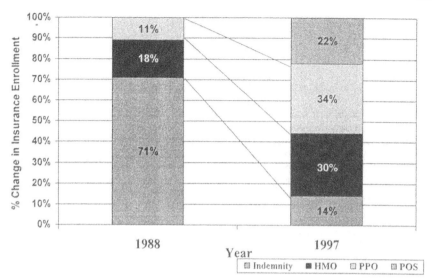

Fig. 1-10. Percentage of U.S. employees enrolled in types of health plans from 1988 to 1997. Source: KPMG Survey of Employer Sponsored Health Benefits—1997.

teams of health care providers who focus on care plans and not individual units of service. Coupled with Americans' increased life span and continued longevity, osteoporosis is a costly and escalating public health problem. If left unchecked, its future costs in money, mortality, and morbidity will be an enormous drain on our resources. The overriding issue is not whether Americans will spend restricted health care resources on osteoporosis, but the issue is how much will we spend and at what stage of life will we spend it. Will it be to prolong life, however frail and debilitated? Or, will it be to enhance and sustain an active and productive life?

SUGGESTED READING

Ankjaer-Jensen A, Johnell O: Prevention of osteoporosis: Cost-effectiveness of different pharmaceutical treatments. Osteoporosis Int 6:26–275, 1996.

Brennan NJ, Caplan GA: Attitudes of osteoporosis and hormone replacement therapy among elderly women. Osteoporosis Int 9:139–141, 1999.

Ferris AK, Wyszewianski L: Quality of ambulatory care for the elderly: Formulating evaluation criteria. Health Care Financing Rev 12:31–38, 1990.

Fox PD, Fama T: Managed care and the elderly: Performance and potential. Generations 22:31–41, 1996.

Gage B: The history and growth of medicare managed care. Generations 22:11–18, 1998.

Goldsmith JC, Goran MJ, Nackel JG: Managed care comes of age. Healthcare Forum J 38(5):14–24, 1995.

Greenspan SL, Maitland-Ramsey L, Myers E: Classification of osteoporosis in the elderly is dependent on site-specific analysis. Calcified Tissue Int 58:409–414, 1996.

Heaney RP: Bone mass, bone loss, and osteoporosis. Ann Intern Med 128:313–314, 1998.

Hunt AH, Repa-Eschen L: Assessment of learning needs of registered nurses for osteoporosis education. Orthop Nursing 17(6):55–60, 1998.

Johnell O, Gullberg P, Kanis JA, Allander E, Elffors L, Dequeker J, Dilsen G, Gennari CA, Vaz AL, Lyritis G, Massuoli G, Miravet L, Passeri M, Cano RP, Rapado A, Ribot C: Risk factors for hip fracture in european women: The MEDOS Study, Bone Miner, 10:1802–1815, 1995.

Kramer AM, Steiner JF, Schlenker RE, Eilertsen TB, Hrincevich CA, Tropea DA, Ahmad LA, Eckhoff DG: Outcomes and costs after hip fracture and stroke. JAMA, 277:396–404, 1997.

Lau EMC, Ho SC, Leung S, and Woo J: Osteoporosis in Asia: Crossing the Frontiers. Singapore: World Scientific Publishing, 1997.

Looker AC, Johnston CC Jr, Wahner HW, Dunn WL, Calvo MS, Harris TB, Heyse SP, Lindsay RL: Prevalence of low femoral bone density in older U.S. women from NHANES III. J Bone Miner 10:796–802, 1995.

Lyritis GP, and the MEDOS Study Group: Epidemiology of hip fracture: The MEDOS Study. Osteoporosis Int 3:S11–S15, 1996.

Medicare Program: Medicare coverage of and payment for bone mass measurements. Federal Register 63:34320–34328, 1998.

Melton LJ, Chrischilles EA, Cooper C, Lane AW, Riggs BL: How many women have osteoporosis? J Bone Miner 7:1005–1010, 1992.

Miller P, Bonnick S, Rosen C et al: Guidelines for the clinical utilization of bone mass measurements in the adult population. Calcified Tissue Int 57:251–252, 1995.

Newton KM: The physician's role in women's decision making about hormone replacement therapy. Obset Gynecol Arch Intern Med 92:580–584, 1998.

Ray NF, Chan JK, Thamer M, Melton III LJ: Medical expenditures for the treatment of osteoporotic fractures in the United States in 1995: Report from the National Osteoporosis Foundation. J Bone Miner 12:24–35, 1997.

Reeve J, and the EPOS Study Group: The European Prospective Osteoporosis Study. Osteoporosis Int 3:S16–S19, 1996.

Ribot C, Tremollieres F, Pouilles, JM: Can we predict women with low bone mass using clinical risk factors? Am J Med 98(Suppl. 2A):52–55, 1995.

Riggs B, Melton LJ III: The worldwide problem of osteoporosis: Insights afforded by epidemiology. Bone 17:S505–S511, 1995.

Rubin SM, Cummings SR: Results of bone densitometry affect women's decisions about taking measures to prevent fractures. Ann Intern Med 116:990–995, 1992.

Silverman SL: Effects of bone density information on decisions about hormone replacement therapy: A randomized trial. Obstet Gynecol 89:321–325, 1997.

Stock JL, Waud CE, Coderre MS, Overdorf JH, Janikas BS, Heinilouma KM, Morris MA: Clinical reporting to primary care physicians leads to increased use and understanding of bone densitometry and affects the management of osteoporosis. Ann Intern Med 218:996–999, 1998.

Suarez-Almazor M, Homik JE, Messina D, Davis P: Attitudes and beliefs of family physicians and gynecologists in relation to the prevention and treatment of osteoporosis, J Bone Miner, 12:1100–1107, 1997.

Terry P: How mature is your organization's prevention effort? Four states of managed care health promotion. Healthcare Forum J 41(5):54–58, 1998.

U.S. Government, Health Care Financing Administration (HCFA), HHS: Medicare program: Medicare coverage of and payments for bone mass measurements. Fed Register, Rules Regul 63:34320–34328, 1998.

U.S. Congress, Office of Technology Assessment: Effectiveness and Costs of Osteoporosis Screening and Hormone Replacement Therapy, Volume 1: Cost-Effectiveness Analysis, OTA-BP-H-160, Washington DC: U.S. Government Printing Office, August 1995.

2 Effects of Aging on Bone Structure and Metabolism

Roberto Pacifici

Louis V. Avioli

Osteoporosis of the senile or postmenopausal variety is defined as a skeletal disorder in which the absolute amount of bone is decreased relative to that of younger, or menstruating, individuals although the remaining bone is normal in chemical composition. Symptomatic senile or postmenopausal osteoporosis syndromes are classically considered to result from the universal loss of bone that normally attends senescence in both sexes. Although comparable decrements in the functional capacity of the heart, lungs, muscle, kidney, and neural tissue also attend the aging process, the decrease in bone mass often results in fractures and immobilization in the aged individual, which requires significant hospitalization time and expenditures, and often marked inactivity and morbidity. Spinal osteoporosis and osteoarthritis (osteoarthrosis) are common findings in elderly populations. However, these disorders represent two distinct disease entities, which are uncommon in the same individual.

Remarkably little is known regarding the underlying pathological process(es) that undermine matrix and cellular aspects of skeletal tissue in the aging, fracture-prone female, although there is a unanimity of opinion that skeletal mass normally decreases with age (Fig. 2-1). It has been suggested that this age-related loss of bone is an appropriate consequence of senescence, simply reflecting an age-dependent dysfunction(s) of bone cellular activity. Bone growth, modeling, and remodeling in the prepubescent years, and the remodeling that continues following ultimate skeletal maturation and epiphyseal closure result from a cybernetic interplay between osteoblast-controlled bone formation and osteoclast-osteocyte modulated bone resorption. A discordant cybernetic "couple" between the osteoblast-osteoclast

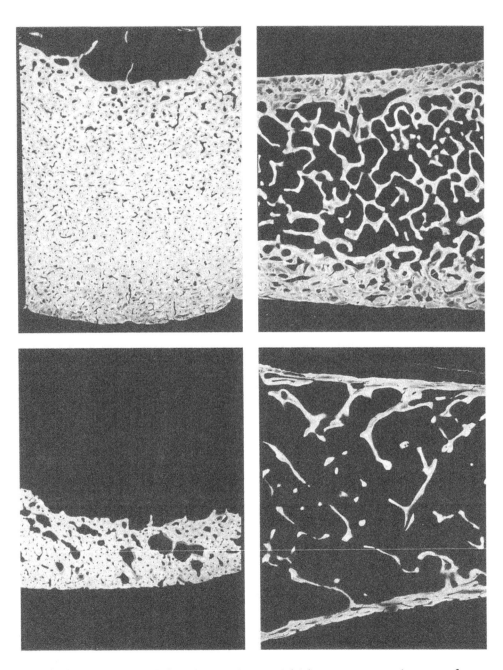

Fig. 2-1. Cortical (top left) and trabecular (top right) bone components in a young female. Compare cortical (bottom left) and trabecular (bottom right) bone in an elderly female. Note the marked decrease in cortical bone content in the elderly female (bottom left) with bone resorption *within the cortical bone* in addition to loss of interconnecting trabeculae in the elderly female (bottom right). Trabecular bone specimens were obtained from iliac crest biopsies. Cortical bone specimens were otained from femoral bone. (Courtesy of J. Jowsey.)

cellular components and an accumulation of mast cells, which probably stimulate bone resorption via secreted "humors," may all contribute to the progressive loss of bone characteristic of the aging process. Because the incidence and prevalence rates of hip fractures in the world at large varies considerably, a variety of other hypothesis have been advanced to explain these differences. These include genetic predisposition and race, latitude and degree of sunlight exposure, physical activity, excessive alcohol, caffeine, nicotine, low calcium intake, and nutritionally inadequate diets.

The skeleton approximates 15–17% of body weight and 80% is composed of cortical bone, the primary component of the extremities or appendicular skeleton. The remaining 20% of skeletal mass is accounted for by trabecular or cancellous bone which, because it is 3–4 times metabolically more active than cortical bone, responds more rapidly to factors or diseases that adversely effect the skeleton. When epiphyseal closure and longitudinal growth of the skeleton are complete, bone turnover and remodeling continues at similar rates. Ultimately, both cortical and trabecular bone mass decrease with advancing years albeit at different rates. Rates of bone loss also depend on sex and race, associated disease processes, relative degrees of gonadal failure, as well as the age when gonadal deficiency occurs. For example, bone mass in active adolescent girls is not only affected by the absence of estrogen exposure, but even the slightest ovulatory disturbances, such as anovulatory cycles and cycles with short luteal phases, result in accelerated spinal bone loss syndromes (Fig. 2-2). Timing of puberty is also an important determinant of peak bone density in men, since men with a history of delayed puberty have decreased bone density in the appendicular and axial skeleton in later life. It should be recognized that in men aged 50–89 years a direct relationship exists between bone mineral density and circulating bioavailable estrogens.

Despite reported beneficial effects of estrogen replacement therapy in postmenopausal patients with fractures and osteoporosis, the relationship between bone loss and circulating ovarian steroids in the elderly postmenopausal female and individual susceptibility to estrogen deficiency is still ill-defined. It has been suggested that reduced amounts of endogenous estrogens may contribute to the greater loss of urinary calcium and more frequent occurrence of osteoporosis in slender postmenopausal women. In favor of this hypothesis are the observations that obese postmenopausal women are less likely to develop rapid bone demineralization and crush fractures than slender women of similar ages, and those that demonstrate that circulating estrone and estradiol levels as well as the peripheral conversion of androstenedione are reduced in slender women in comparison to obese subjects. Isolated observations of lower vaginal maturation values in postmenopausal women with osteoporosis compared to those without osteoporosis have also led to the suggestion that estrogen deficiency is more severe in the former. Lower circulating levels of estrone and androstenedione have been reported for osteoporotic females by some investigators,

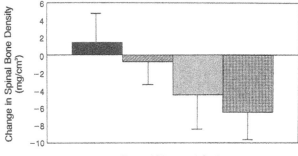

Type of Menstrual Cycle

Fig. 2-2. Mean (± SD) change in spinal bone density, as measured by computed to-mography, in relation to the menstrual cycle experience of 66 normal premenopausal women studied for 1 year. The 13 women with luteal phases of consistently normal length (10-16 days) during the year (solid bar) and the 12 women with a short luteal phase during only one cycle (hatched bar) had bone-density values that were significantly different from those of the 28 women who had more than one cycle with a short luteal phase (stippled bar) or of the 13 women who had anovulatory cycles (dotted bar). T=5.37, $p<.0001$. (Reproduced from Prior JC et al: N Engl J Med 323:1221-1227, 1990. Copyright © 1990 Massachusetts Medical Society. All rights reserved.)

while others using age-matched controls observed similar levels of circulating total estrogens in postmenopausal women with or without osteoporosis. No significant differences in androstenedione levels were seen when comparing women with accelerated bone demineralization to those with decreased rates of bone loss. Most would agree that the loss of appendicular bone observed in postmenopausal women results primarily from the loss of estrogens. Although the biological response to this insult in skeletal tissues is still ill-defined at best, it is becoming increasingly obvious that a variety of cytokines which regulate osteoclastic bone resorption such as interleukin 1, interleukin 6, tumor necrosis factor, macrophage colony stimulating factor (M-CSF) and the newly discovered osteoprotegerin ligand (OPGL) are contributory in this regard. These observations are consistent with others demonstrating that higher circulating levels of the interleukin 6 cytokine which occur with ovarian deficiency (Fig. 2-3) actually predict disability onset in elderly individuals.

As illustrated in Fig. 2-4, the "calciotropic" hormones PTH, calcitonin, and vitamin D_3 metabolites [25-(OH)D_3 and 1,25-(OH)$_2D_3$] normally function to maintain exquisite cybernetic control over calcium absorption, circulating ionized calcium, and bone remodeling. It is becoming increasingly apparent that blood PTH levels increase with age and that supranormal levels occur in some elderly patients with symptomatic osteoporosis. The age-related rise in PTH has been attributed to an associated age-related decrease in renal function, poor dietary calcium intake, defective adaptive renal function,

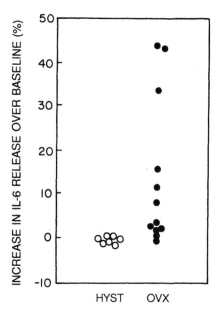

Fig. 2-3. Increments in interleukin 6 (IL-6) secretion by peripheral blood mononuclear cells in women 40 days following oophorectomy. Hyst denotes control subjects with hysterectomy and no oophorectomy; ovx, oophorectomized individuals. (Adapted with permission from G. Pioli et al., 1992, Clinical Science 83:503, 1992. © the Biochemical Society and the Medical Research Society.)

and defective absorptive mechanisms resulting from impaired hepatic and renal hydroxylation of vitamin D and 25-(OH)D (Fig. 2-4). The contribution of this "senescent" hyperparathyroid syndrome to the normal age-related decrease in bone mass, and to the crush fracture osteoporotic syndrome, is controversial. It appears naive, however, to ignore observations that the rate of bone loss in postmenopausal women is greater in those with reduced dietary calcium intake and higher blood levels of PTH, and others defining relationships between progressive increments in circulating PTH and urinary cyclic adenosine monophosphate (cAMP) with age, and the steadily declining intake of calcium in women, which in the United States is significantly less than the recommended daily allowance (RDA). The primary secretagogue for PTH is any change in circulating ionized calcium due to a perturbation in dietary intake, defective intestinal absorption, or increased excretion of calcium, each of which can deplete the circulating ionized calcium pool (Fig. 2-4). Of note in this regard are reports defining a tendency toward elevated PTH levels in elderly patients with vertebral osteoporosis and hip fractures.

There is currently little information regarding seasonal and/or age-related changes in blood levels of all vitamin D metabolites. It appears that sunlight

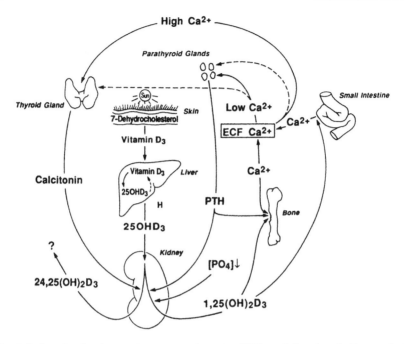

Fig. 2-4. Feedback relations between calcitonin, PTH, and the vitamin D_3 metabolic pathway. (Solid lines represent stimulatory activities, and dashed lines represent suppressive influences.) Note that the bioactivation of 25-(OH)D_3 by the kidney is stimulated by PTH as well as the tendency to low circulating phosphate concentrations ($[PO_4]\downarrow$). The resulting 1,25-(OH)$_2D_3$ functions primarily to increase the intestinal absorption of calcium. To date, the biological activity of the 24,25-(OH)$_2D_3$ in humans is still conjectural at best.

can influence the levels of 25-(OH)D_3 with low values characteristic of winter seasons. Certain observations suggest that synthesis of 25-(OH)D_3 and 1,25-(OH)$_2D_3$ decreases with age. The apparent impaired conversion of 25-(OH)D_3 to 1,25-(OH)$_2D_3$ has been attributed by some to a decrease in factors that abnormally stimulate the converting enzyme, 25-(OH)D_3 1α-hydroxylase, which normally is responsive to PTH. The osteoporosis and age-related decrease in intestinal calcium absorption has been attributed to low 1,25-(OH)$_2D_3$, as well as marginally low levels of circulating 25-(OH)D_3. These acquired, subtle vitamin D deficiencies contribute to the osteomalacic syndrome and progressive increments in the incidence of femoral neck fractures, which characterize clinical profiles of elderly osteoporotic populations. The role of calcitonin in the day-to-day control of skeletal remodeling processes in humans is still uncertain. In some studies, calcitonin levels are lower in females than in males, with blood levels of this hormone appearing to decrease with advancing age. Both low and normal calcitonin levels have been observed in some patients with accelerated osteoporotic syndromes. Finally, it has also been speculated that a lifelong relative deficiency of calcitonin in some women could play a role in age- and sex-related bone loss, particularly during the estrogen-deficient postmenopausal years. Increments in blood calcitonin levels which have been observed in some estrogen-treated females are considered consistent with this hypothesis.

The fundamental etiology and pathogenesis of the progressive loss of bone in the elderly, when hormones such as estrogens and androgens are no longer pivotal in controlling bone remodeling and the cybernetic coupling between the bone forming osteoblasts and bone resorbing osteoclasts, are still conjectural at best. According to the quantum concept of bone remodeling, all gains or losses of bone are the result of focal imbalance, during individual remodeling cycles between the depth of a cavity in bone formed as a result of erosion by osteoclast cells and the thickness of new bone deposited in the cavity by osteoblast cells. A decline in the wall thickness of the cavity with aging is well established and attributed to "osteoblastic failure." Bone marrow stromal cells have long been considered the source of osteoprogenitor cells although heretofore the data from humans was lacking to substantiate this hypothesis. Pluripotential stromal stem cells in the bone marrow compartment can differentiate into fibroblasts, adipocytes, reticular cells, or osteoprogenitor cells. Renewal of the osteoblast population at the bone surface is thought to occur via differentiation of osteoprogenitor cells along the osteoblast lineage. Stromal cells may also play a dual role in new bone formation by providing "osteotropic factor(s)," which either promote or inhibit osteoblast DNA synthesis and proliferation. Stromal cells also synthesize many of the cytokines (e.g., OPGL and M-CSF), which define the lineage of primitive osteogenic precursor cells. A summary of key osteoclastogenic cytokines and of the cell required for inducing osteoclast formation is shown in Fig. 2-5.

Although the aging process per se might conceivably affect a variety of these stromal cell "activities," one possibility is that the bone marrow supply of osteoprogenitor cells decreases as a consequence of aging. It is noteworthy however, that despite an age-related decrease of active hemopoietic tissue in the bone marrow, there is no substantial decrease in the number of peripheral blood elements in the elderly population because of an increased proliferation of committed granulopoietic stem cells in hypoplastic areas of bone marrow. Elevations in serum lysozyme activity in healthy, aged individuals is also consistent with the contention that total granulocytic mass is not diminished in old age. Growth stimulatory or factors normally secreted by human bone marrow cells may be altered during the aging process resulting in diminished proliferation of osteoblasts. In this regard in vitro studies reveal that bone marrow stromal cells produce factors that stimulate osteoblast proliferation. In addition, bone marrow transplanted from aged animal into young animals induces bone loss while bone loss in aged animals can be reversed or prevented by transplantation of young bone marrow. Thus, it is still unclear whether age-related osteoblastic failure reflects a

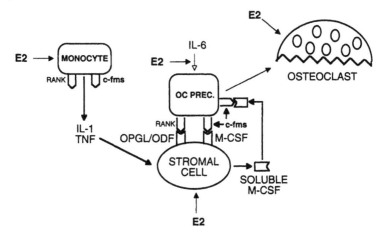

Fig. 2-5. Cells and cytokines essential for osteoclast formation. Osteoclasts arise from hematopoietic precursors of the monocytic lineage which express the M-CSF receptor c-fms and the OPGL receptor RANK. These cells secrete interleukin 1 (IL-1) and tumor necrosis factor (TNF), two factors capable of inducing the production of M-CSF (both soluble and membrane bound) by bone marrow stromal cells. OPGL and M-CSF induce proliferation of monocytes and their differentiation into mature osteoclasts. E2 represses osteoclast formation by blocking the monocytic production of IL-1 and TNF and by decreasing the stromal cell production of OPGL, M-CSF, and IL-6. OPG, osteoprotegerin; OPGL, OPG ligand; M-CSF, macrophage colony stimulating factor; RANK, OPGL receptor; c-fms, M-CSF receptor.

decreased number of mature osteoblasts, an impairment in the proliferation, recruitment, and differentiation of marrow osteoprogenitor cells, or a defect in osteotropic factors produced by the immature osteoprogenitor stromal cells.

SUMMARY AND CONCLUSIONS

Analyses of age-related bone loss patterns in females reveal (1) progressive loss of axial (trabecular) bone mass, which begins sometime in the third decade; and (2) a decrease in appendicular (cortical) bone mass beginning in the fifth decade with an accelerated rate of decline during the sixth and early part of the seventh decade. Although those factors that initiate and/or perpetuate this age-bone loss phenomenon are still ill-defined, they result in an "uncoupling" of the cybernetic interplay between osteoblast-controlled bone formation and osteoclastic-osteocytic modulated bone resorption with the latter predominating. The "uncoupling" must be greater in aging females than males since the incidence of nontraumatic skeletal fractures in the elderly is greater in the former. Differential patterns of trabecular and cortical bone loss may result in at least two distinct osteoporotic syndromes: one is characterized by accelerated and proportionate loss of trabecular bone and an increased incidence of vertebral or Colles' fractures in the immediate postmenopausal years; the other is characterized by a proportionate loss of both cortical and trabecular bone resulting in fractures of the hip and pelvis in the seventh and eighth decades. Although the hormonal milieu that modulates these age-related bone loss syndromes is still conjectural, and currently based only on cross-sectional studies, we must consider the following: (1) gradual increments in parathyroid hormone secretion with age, possibly as a result of chronic dietary calcium deficiency and age-related decreases in the intestinal absorptive capacity for elemental calcium; (2) lower circulating calcitonin values in females than males with a limited secreting capacity following food ingestion of calcium enriched diets; (3) decreased dietary vitamin D intake and sunlight exposure with age with associated decrements in circulating 25-(OH)D$_3$; and (4) decreased ovarian function alteration in the circulating estradiol–estrone balance; and (5) an increase in the production of bone resorbing cytokines. One can reasonably assume that the following sequence of events either initiate and/or perpetuate bone loss in the aging population: premenopausal dietary calcium deficiency → mild and progressive increments in PTH secretion → mild alterations in the PTH–estrogen balance → subtle increments in bone loss; ovarian failure → decreased circulatory estrogens → exaggerated skeletal response to PTH–estrogen imbalance and stimulation of bone resorbing cytokines → more rapid bone loss. This coupled series of PTH–estrogen–bone interplay should obviously be more destructive to the female skeleton: (1) at any age males ingest more calcium than females and are less likely to require parathyroid stimulation and bone resorption to maintain homeostasis; (2) not only are calcitonin levels higher in males than females, but the secretory capacity for this bone sparing hormone following food ingestion in males is apparently greater than that of females; and (3) gonadal function in the male with regard to testosterone production proceeds in a relatively normal fashion well into the seventh and eighth decades. Age-related alterations in circulating 1,25-(OH)$_2$D$_3$ due either to limited reserve of the renal 1α-hydroxylase enzyme, which converts 25-(OH)D$_3$ to 1,25-(OH)$_2$D$_3$, could perpetuate this cycle by the following mechanism: further decreasing dietary calcium absorption → accelerated increments in PTH → greater distortion of the PTH–estrogen ratio → accelerated bone resorption. Additional insult to bone mineralization conditioned by decreases in blood 25-(OH)D$_3$ in selected populations probably adds an osteomalacic component to the progressive osteoporotic process. Finally, we must consider the fact that the decrease in the osteoblastic mediated "bone formation" observed with advancing age in the elderly skeleton may result from acquired deficiencies in either the mobilization of immature marrow osteoprogenitor stem cells and/or in their conversion to mature bone forming osteoblasts.

SUGGESTED READING

Arlot MR, Delmas PH, Chappard D, Meunier PJ: Trabecular and endocortical bone remodeling in postmenopausal osteoporosis: Comparison with normal postmenopausal women. Osteoporosis Int 1:41–49, 1990.

Armamento-Villareal R, Villareal DT, Avioli LV, Civitelli R: Estrogen status and heredity are major determinants of premenopausal bone mass. J Clin Invest 90:2462–2471, 1992.

Bianco P, Robey PG: Perspective: Diseases of bone and the stromal cell lineage. J Bone Miner Res 14:336–341, 1999.

Dhuper S, Warren MP, Brooks-Gunn J, Fox R: Effects of hormonal status on bone density in adolescent girls. J Clin Endocrinol Metab 71:1083–1088, 1990.

Ettinger B, Genant HK, Cann CE: Postmenopausal bone loss is prevented by treatment with low-dosage estrogen with calcium. Ann Intern Med 106:40–45, 1987.

Ferrucci L, Harris TB, Guralnik JM, Tracy RP, Corti MC, Cohen HJ, Penninx B, Pahor M, Wallace R, Havlik RJ: Serum IL-6 level and the development of disability in older persons. JAGS 47:639–646, 1999.

Finkelstein JS, Neer RM, Biller BMK, Crawford JD, Klibanski A: Osteopenia in men with a history of delayed puberty. N Engl J Med 326:600–604, 1992.

Gambacciani M, Spinetti A, De Simone L, Cappagli B, Maffei S, Taponeco F, Fioretti P: The relative contributions of menopause and aging to postmenopausal vertebral osteopenia. J Clin Endocrinol Metab 77:1148–1151, 1993.

Gilsanz V, Roe TF, Mora S, Costin G, Goodman WG: Changes in vertebral bone density in black girls and white girls during childhood puberty. N Engl J Med 325:1597–1600, 1991.

Greendale GA, Edelstein S, Barrett-Connor E: Endogenous sex steroids and bone mineral density in older women and men: The Rancho Bernardo study. J Bone Miner Res 12:1833–1843, 1997.

Hagino H, Yamamoto K, Teshima R, Kishimoto H, Kagawa T: Radial bone mineral changes in pre- and postmenopausal healthy Japanese women: Cross-sectional and longitudinal studies. J Bone Miner Res 7:147–159, 1992.

Halloran BP, Portale AA, Lonegan ET, Morris RC Jr: Production and metabolic clearance of 1,25-dihydroxyvitamin D in men: Effect of advancing age. J Clin Endocrinol Metab 70:318–322, 1990.

Haynesworth SE, Goshima J, Goldberg VM, Caplan AI: Characterization of cells with osteogenic potential from human marrow. Bone 13:81–88, 1992.

Hill PA, Tumber A, Papaioannou S, Meikle MC: The cellular actions of interleukin-11 on bone resorption *in vitro*. Endocrinology (Baltimore) 139:1564–1572, 1998.

Jacques PF, Felson DT, Tucker KL, Mahnken B, Wilson PWF, Rosenberg IH, Rush D: Plasma 25-hydroxyvitamin D and its determinants in an elderly population sample. Am J Clin Nutr 66:929–936, 1997.

Khosla S: Editorial: Idiopathic Osteoporosis—Is the osteoblast to blame? J Clin Endocrinol Metab 82:2792–2793, 1997.

Long MW, Ashcraft EK, Normalle D, Mann KG: Age-related phenotypic alterations in populations of purified human bone precursor cells. J Gerontol 54A:B54–B62, 1999.

Malina RM: Skeletal maturation rate in North American Negro and white children. Nature (London) 223:1075, 1969.

Manolagas SC, Jilka RL: Bone marrow, cytokines and bone remodeling. Emerging insights into the pathogenesis of osteoporosis. N Engl J Med 332:305–311, 1995.

Mazess RB: Bone mineral in Vilcabamba, Ecuador. Am J Roentgenol 130:671–674, 1978.

Meier DE, Orwoll ES, Jones JM: Marked disparity between trabecular and cortical bone loss with age in healthy men. Ann Intern Med 101:605–612, 1984.

Melton LJ III, Khosla S, Atkinson EJ O'Fallon WM, Riggs BL: Relationship of bone turnover to bone density and fractures. J Bone Miner Res 12:1083–1091, 1997.

Moore M, Bracker M, Sartoris D, Saltman P, Strause L: Long-term estrogen replacement therapy in postmenopausal women sustains vertebral bone mineral density. J Bone Miner Res 5:659–664, 1990.

Pacifici R: Estrogen, cytokines, and pathogenesis of postmenopausal osteoporosis. J Bone Miner Res 11:1043–1051, 1996.

Pacifici R, Rifas L, Teitelbaum S, Slatopolsky E, McCracken R, Bergfeld M, Lee W, Avioli LV, Peck WA: Spontaneous release of interleukin 1 from human blood monocytes reflects bone formation in idiopathic osteoporosis. Proc Natl Acad Sci USA 84:4616–4620, 1987.

Pocock NA, Eisman JA, Mazess RB, Sambrook PN, Yeates MG, Freund J: Bone mineral density in Australia compared with the United States. J Bone Miner Res 3:601–603, 1988.

Prior JC, Vigna YM, Schechter MT, Burgess AE: Spinal bone loss and ovulatory disturbances. N Engl J Med 323:1221–1227, 1990.

Ravn P, Rix M, Andreassen H, Clemmesen B, Bidstrup M, Gunnes M: High bone turnover is associated with low bone mass and spinal fracture in postmenopausal women. Calcif Tissue Int 60:255–260, 1997.

Ribot C, Tremollieres F, Pouilles JM, Louvet JP, Guiraud R: Influence of the menopause and aging on spinal density in French women. Bone Miner 5:89–97, 1988.

Rodan GA: Introduction to bone biology. Bone 13:S3–S6, 1992.

Stamp TCB, Round JM: Seasonal changes in human plasma levels of 25-hydroxyvitamin D. Nature (London) 247:563–565, 1974.

Takano-Yamamoto T, Rodan GA: Direct effects of 17-estradiol on trabecular bone in ovariectomized rats. Proc Natl Acad Sci USA 87:2172–2176, 1990.

Webb AR, Kline L, Holick MF: Influence of season and latitude on the cutaneous synthesis of vitamin D_3: Exposure to winter sunlight in Boston and Edmonton will not promote vitamin D_3 synthesis in human skin. J Clin Endocrinol Metab 67:373–378, 1988.

Yoshimura N: Incidence of fast bone losers and factors affecting changes in bone mineral density: A cohort study in a rural Japenese community. Bone Miner Metab 14:171–177, 1996.

3 The Genetics of Osteoporosis

Clifford J. Rosen

INTRODUCTION

The prevalence of osteoporosis has increased dramatically since the late 1980s. Part of this can be traced to longer life spans and a greater awareness of the disease. In addition, a new working definition of osteoporosis based purely on a bone mineral density less than 2.5 standard deviations from young normal greatly expanded the number of people with this disease. The very strong association of bone mass with fracture risk has also led to the use of bone density as a surrogate phenotype for osteoporosis. Thus the development and utilization of bone mass measurements has not only made the diagnosis of this disorder easier but also opened up the possibility that osteoporosis may be a heritable disorder. In this chapter I will focus on the evidence to support the thesis that there is heritability for the bone mass phenotype and the issues which surround the current search for "bone density" genes.

BONE DENSITY AS A PHENOTYPE FOR OSTEOPOROSIS

Numerous epidemiologic studies have defined an inverse relationship between bone mineral density (BMD) at any skeletal site and subsequent risk for an osteoporotic fracture. Indeed, for every 1 standard deviation decline in BMD, there is an approximately 2-fold greater risk of spine or hip fracture. Moreover, there is no threshold effect, so that the lower the BMD the greater is the relative risk (RR). And this relationship is maintained even when age, sex, and body mass index are kept constant. This association has permitted a more rapid and accurate assessment of fracture risk in younger individuals without apparent disease. It has also allowed investigators to examine the heritability of this disease without waiting for a fracture to become clinically apparent.

Bone mineral density is an ideal phenotype for genetic studies. At any site by any measurement tool [computed tomography (CT), dual-energy X-ray absorptiometry (DXA), single-energy X-ray absorptiometry (SXA), ultrasound] BMD is a quantitative trait. This means that expression of a trait in a given individual can be described numerically, based on an appropriate form of measurement. Quantitative traits are also called "continuous," in contrast to qualitative traits that are expressed in the form of distinct phenotypes such as eye color. Continuous traits in humans include blood pressure, IQ, musical talent, height, and longevity. These phenotypes are usually distributed in a Gaussian manner with symmetrical variation around the mean. This allows for a wide range of values in a given population. Indeed, this is the case for BMD, whether it is in a small cohort of postmenopausal women or the entire population of Canada.

Although quantitative traits can be easily measured, these phenotypes are almost always a function of multiple genetic influences. Occasionally a single mutation in a given polymorphic locus can give rise to continuous variation with a population. However, that condition, or a mutant allele at a single locus leading to variable expressivity, is rarely noted in the human population. Instead, a continuous phenotype is synonymous with multiple genetic interactions. For example, height is a polygenic trait defined by numerous genetic determinants, some which are additive, and some that alter the expression of other genes. Similarly bone mass is a complex trait characterized by multiple genetic determinants, pleiotropy, epistasis, nonlinear associations, and multiple variants.

Continuous variation in the expression of a trait can also be due to environmental factors which interact with specific genes. The latter include hormonal, pharmacological, environmental, and nutritional determinants. The role of these factors in defining bone mineral density across the life span of a given individual has been defined and emphasized in many studies over the last three decades. In particular, acute and/or chronic estrogen deficiency, poor dietary calcium and vitamin D, and exogenous glucocorticoids predispose individuals to low bone mass. Several lines of evidence suggest that heritable factors may be at least as important as environmental factors in defining the bone density phenotype. This ultimately means that most osteoporotic fractures will prove to be a function of several genetic factors. Since bone density is an appropriate phenotype for osteoporotic risk, and is accessible, quantifiable, and reproducible, the search for "bone density" genes has become very focused. However, it should be noted that BMD is not the only phenotype which could be used in defining genetic determinants of osteoporosis. For example, one could choose bone size, a biochemical marker of bone turnover (e.g., osteocalcin), or calcaneal ultrasound attenuation as surrogate markers for osteoporosis. Even more obvious of a choice would be the appearance of an osteoporotic fracture. The final common denominator of osteoporosis is clearly a fracture. These events, however, are usually not manifested until late in life. Moreover, spine fractures can be difficult to diagnose and require X-ray confirmation. Therefore, assessing large populations at risk would become much more difficult. On the other hand, accuracy, ease of use, and the continuous nature of bone mass measurements make DXA an obvious choice to screen for genetic determinants.

EVIDENCE FOR HERITABILITY OF BONE DENSITY

What Is Heritability?

The first step in establishing genetic determinants of any disease state is defining the heritability of the phenotype under study. Heritability is a quantitative estimate of the fraction of the phenotypic variation that is the result of genetic differences among individuals. Mathematically, it is defined as a ratio of the fraction of phenotypic variance due to genetic differences divided by the total phenotypic variance observed for a given trait. The heritability (H) value for a given trait depends on the specific population and the environment in which the variation occurs. Although often used synonymously with correlation, heritability represents a numerical attempt to quantify the genetic variation for a particular phenotype. It requires knowledge of the environmental variability. Simple correlational analysis can only provide an estimate of the variance that can be attributed to an independent variable in relation to the dependent variable (e.g., calcium intake independent versus bone mineral density dependent).

Evidence That Bone Mass Is Heritable

Bone mineral density at any age is a function of the rate of bone acquisition during adolesence and the rate of bone loss after menopause and during later life. Current projections suggest that more than 60% of the variance in BMD at any time in an individual's life is related to their peak bone mass. Hence, factors that affect peak BMD have received tremendous attention. Several lines of evidence suggest that much of variance in peak bone mass relates to genetic factors. For a number of years, investigators have known that a strong family history of osteoporosis is associated with a greater risk of fracture. Data from the SOF (Study of Osteoporotic Fractures) more recently confirmed that a maternal history of hip fracture is an independent risk factor for future fracture. Studies in family members have also been revealing. Earlier work showed strong correlations between mothers and daughters for hip BMD. Subsequent examination revealed that monozygotic twins had nearly identical BMD values, whereas dizygotic twins had significant variability. More recent analyses have calculated the heritability of BMD based on the twin model. Using mono- and dizygotic twins, H was determined as the ratio of the difference in variance between dizygotic and monozygotic BMD divided by the variance for dizygotics: $(VDZ - VMZ)/(VDZ)$. On the basis of these and other studies, the H for spine or hipbone mass is estimated to be between 0.4 and 0.5. Therefore, much of the variance in peak bone mass can be explained by genetic factors.

Studies in animal models have also provided strong evidence to support the heritability of bone density. For healthy inbred strains of mice peak bone mass may differ by as much as 50%, and it is estimated that as much as 80% of the variability in murine bone density measured by peripheral quantitative computed tomography (pQCT) is related to genetic determinants. In baboons, Mahaney, Rogers, and others (1997) have demonstrated moderately strong heritability for bone density of the spine and hip. Furthermore, by use of multigenerational pedigrees this group found significant genetic correlations for BMD between three vertebrae but no genetic correlations between spine and forearm BMD (despite a relatively strong phenotypic correlation between sites). These data, and other preliminary studies in mice, support the hypothesis that bone mass is heritable, and that various skeletal sites may be affected by different genes.

MEANS OF DEFINING GENETIC DETERMINANTS OF BONE MASS IN HUMANS

A complete understanding of the genetic basis for variation in osteoporosis risk should include information describing the number of loci exerting influence, the magnitude and nature of the effects of these loci, and the patterns of interactions among genes and between genes and the environment. In order to begin that process, several different approaches have been undertaken. These include twin studies, genetic association analyses in unrelated populations, studies of known mutations in genes related to bone metabolism, family linkage studies, and combination studies involving initial linkage assessments followed by whole genome scanning in sib-pairs or large populations. Twin studies have been used to confirm the familial aggregation of osteoporosis, and the heritability of BMD. However, the number of subjects is limited and the cost is high. Furthermore, there are methodological limitations inherent in twin studies which make conclusions about specific genetic effects on traits somewhat tenuous. Genetic association studies are easier to perform and remain the most popular although the information obtained must be considered within the context of the methodology. In association studies, a polymorphic region in or near a "candidate" gene is typed for its various alleles within a given population. Subsequently, the frequency of a specific genotype and its relationship to BMD is noted.

The first polymorphism to be extensively studied was in the vitamin D receptor gene (VDR), where a noncoding region in an intron was found to be highly polymorphic within a population and to be related to BMD both in twins and in a larger cohort from Australia. One particular genotype (BB−, representing the absence of a cut point with a restriction enzyme) was related to not only low BMD but also serum osteocalcin. These data suggested that a polymorphic segment in a nonfunctional region of the VDR gene could affect bone turnover and/or calcium metabolism. Subsequent trials have produced very conflicting results in which some studies have shown absolutely no relationship between those VDR alleles and BMD, whereas others confirmed a relationship. Thus, the strength of any association between VDR alleles and bone mass is uncertain.

Other "candidate" loci have also been studied by association analyses. These include a functional region in the VDR gene, a polymorphic loci of the estrogen receptor gene, a region in the collagen 1A1 gene which is in approximation to a transcriptional regulation site, a dinucleotide repeat in the IGF-I gene, and polymorphic regions in the interleukin-1 gene. All these studies share the same methodology and all have produced somewhat inconsistent results when analyzed by various laboratories. To a small degree, this could be explained by differences in various populations and laboratories. However, it is clear that for association studies to be successful in defining genetic loci, several components are absolutely essential: (1) complete definition of the phenotype under study, (2) recognition of the numerous covariates which influence the phenotype, (3) a large sample size, and (4) knowledge of the population and its variability. Although BMD has been defined as an appropriate phenotype, the other criteria raise questions about the validity of association studies. Indeed, the biggest concern relates to sample size. Studies with less than 500 unrelated subjects are prone to significant sampling error. Hence, information from association studies with presumed candidates has been helpful, although these have not produced consistent genetic "loci" which regulate peak bone mass.

Family studies of inborn errors or mutations that lead to osteoporosis have been another approach undertaken by several groups. Clearly, as noted above, a single gene defect does not cause low bone mass. However, osteogenesis imperfecta is a familial disease characterized by qualitative abnormalities in collagen which lead to severe osteoporosis with multiple fractures and very low bone mineral density. Variants of this disease, either due to incomplete penetrance or other changes, can cause low bone mass and a less severe form of the disease. Recently Spotilla, Prockop, and others (1991) have identified mutations in the Col 1A1 gene which in two families has been associated with an osteoporosis phenotype. Although it is unlikely that single mutations in this gene could cause the wide variation in bone mass among normal individuals, it is possible that this will turn out to be one of many genes which contributes to the osteoporosis phenotype. Indeed, the very recent finding in an association study, that a polymorphism in the Col A1A gene can be related to both BMD and fracture suggests this may be one true candidate loci.

Family linkage studies have been proposed as another way to find "bone density" genes. Analysis of quantitative traits in individuals from large multi-generational families allows the investigator to quantify the effects of individual genes, polygenic backgrounds, and environmental factors on a complex trait. The genetic power of such an approach is derived from the varying degree of genetic similarity for BMD. One of the most successful examples of such a quest has been the elucidation of a high bone mineral density genetic loci. Recker and colleagues (1997) have identified more than 250 members of a family, some of whom have very high bone density. The original observation happened somewhat by chance when high bone mass was noted on plain X-ray films in an individual who sustained multiple trauma but did not suffer any fractures. Subsequently, investigators were able to successfully map a genetic loci on chromosome 11 which is associated with high bone mineral density in several family members. This particular region of chromosome 11 has also been linked to a syndrome of pseudo-ganglioma and low bone mass. Intense efforts to positionally clone this region will ultimately lead to the discovery of the first genetic loci associated with bone mass.

Studies of extended families and sib-pairs without predisposing skeletal conditions has been another approach to defining "bone density" genes. Several groups have recruited large numbers of sib-pairs and have studied both extreme discordant and concordant sibs for BMD. This approach is combined with whole genome scanning to identify potential regions of the genome which map to high or low bone density. This strategy has also been applied to candidate loci previously identified from pure association studies. The region in chromosome 11 previously identified by linkage studies has also been noted to be one determinant of BMD in sib studies. More investigations using this approach are likely to be published in the next several years.

Animal studies have generally supported the observations noted earlier in humans. The BMD phenotype in mice and baboons is polygenic with as many as 20 genes contributing to overall bone density. Several investigators have identified relatively large genomic regions [also called quantitative trait loci (QTLs)] that affect the BMD phenotype in mice. These regions are currently being studied on a functional basis by development of congenic mice (i.e., one loci from a high-density strain introduced into a low-density background) and structurally by fine mapping and positional cloning. Similarly, baboon genotyping has led investigators to examine human candidate loci including that on chromosome 11.

In summary, it is clear that bone density as measured by DXA or other instruments is a suitable phenotype for studying the genetics of osteoporosis. But it is the not the only one. Calcaneal ultrasound, peripheral DXA of the wrist or calcaneus, and peripheral CT all predict fractures with similar accuracy as regular DXA. Hence, more large-scale screening studies with peripheral instruments may improve our chances of finding various genetic determinants. But this trait is polygenic and likely controlled by numerous genes. In addition, there are likely to be significant gene–gene and gene–environment interactions that will complicate interpretation of major genetic loci which will be identified in the next decade. Strategies to find those genes will include the approaches noted above and further studies in animal models.

FUTURE STUDIES

Bone mass is a complex trait characterized by multiple genetic determinants, pleiotropy, epistasis, gene–environmental interactions, nonlinear associations, and multiple variants. Therefore, strategies to define specific genes that regulate this trait will have to be inclusive. Even if those predefined conditions are met, and both linkage and association studies are performed, successful mapping of specific loci is still likely to be exceedingly difficult. For example, there are well-known discrepencies between physical and genetic maps. Moreover, candidate regions are still very large and are susceptible to complex interactions between genes. Finally, positional cloning and fine mapping to identify specific genes requires tremendous time, effort, and support. Despite those concerns, it is clear that much progress has been made in defining the genetic regulation of bone mass. When specific loci or genes are identified, it is conceivable that screening individuals at the greatest risk for low bone density by rapid genetic analysis will occur. Unlike some disorders where genetic screening is not accompanied by specific therapeutic interventions, it is almost certain that the genes which define low bone mass are modifiable by environmental factors such as calcium intake or exercise. Hence, large-scale preventive strategies of adolescents at risk may be hastened with the discovery of the genes which control bone mineral density and osteoporosis risk.

SUGGESTED READING

Beamer WG, Donahue LR, Rosen CJ, Baylink DJ: Genetic variability in adult bone density among inbred strains of mice. Bone 18:397–405, 1996.

Consensus Development Conference 1993: Diagnosis, prophylaxis and treatment of osteoporosis. Am J Med 94:646–649, 1993.

Cummings SR, Black DM, Nevitt MC, Browner WS, Cauley JA, Genant HK, Mascioli SR, Scott JC, Seeley DG, Steiger P, Vogt TM: Appendicular bone density and age predict hip fracture in women. JAMA 263:665–668, 1990.

Gong Y, Vikkula M, Boon L, Liu J, Beighton P, Ramesar R, Peltonen L, Somer H, Hirose T, Dallapicoola B, DePaepe A, Swoboda W, Zabel B, Superti-Furga A,

Steinmann B, Brunner HG, Jans A, Boles RG, Adkins W, van den Boogaard MJ, Olsen BR, Warman ML: Osteoporosis pseudoganglioma syndrome: A disorder affecting skeletal strength and visions is assigned to chromosome region 11q 12–13. Am J Hum Genet 59:146–151, 1996.

Hansen MA, Hassager C, Jensen SB, Christiansen C: Is heritability a risk factor for postmenopausal osteoporosis? J Bone Miner Res 9:1037–1043, 1992.

Jenkins JB: Complex patterns of inheritance. In Jenkins JJ (ed): Human Genetics. New York: Harper Collins, 1990, pp 392–425.

Johnson ML, Gong G, Kimberling W, Recker SM, Kimmel DB, Recker RB: Linkage of a gene causing high bone mass to chromosome 11(11q12–13). Am J Hum Genet 60:1326–1332, 1997.

Morrison NA, Qi JC, Tokiat A, Kelley PJ, Crofts L, Nguyen TV, Sambrook PN, Eisman JA: Prediction of bone density from vitamin D receptor alleles. Nature (London) 367:284–287, 1994.

Pocock NA, Eisman JA, Hopper JL, Yeates MG, Sambrook PN, Eberl S: Genetic determinants of bone mass in adults: A twin study. J Clin Invest 80:706–710, 1987.

Rogers J, Mahaney MC, Beamer WG, Donahue LR, Rosen CJ: Beyond one gene–one disease: Alternative strategies of deciphering genetic determinants of osteoporosis. Calcif Tissue Int 60:225–228, 1997.

Seeman E, Hopper JL, Bach LA, Cooper ME, Parkinson E, McKay J, Jerums G: Reduced bone mass in daughters of women with osteoporosis. N Engl J Med 320:554–558, 1989.

Spotila LD, Constantinou CD, Sereda L, Ganguly A, Riggs BL, Prockop DJ: Mutations in gene for type I procollagen in women with postmenopausal osteoporosis: Evidence for phenotypic and genotypic overlap with mild osteogenesis imperfecta. Proc Natl Acad Sci USA 88:5423–5427, 1991.

Uitterlinden AG, Burger H, Huang Q, Yue F, McGuigan FE, Grant SF, Hofman A, van Leeuwen JP, Pols HA, Ralston SH. Relation of alleles of the collagen type I alpha 1 gene to bone density and the risk of osteoporotic fractures in postmenopausal women. N Engl J Med 338:1016–1021, 1998.

4 Bone Mass Measurement Techniques in Clinical Practice

Barbara B. Sterkel

Paul D. Miller

INTRODUCTION

Radiographs have provided imaging of bone since the turn of the twentieth century, and refinement of radiographic techniques has allowed characterization of bone, cortical and trabecular bone, and bone lesions. One limitation of plain radiography in identifying bone loss is insensitivity. In addition, analog images that characterize routine radiograph procedures do not allow quantification of mineral. Since the early 1960s various techniques have developed that now permit quick, noninvasive, and accurate quantitation of bone mass with essentially no risk or discomfort for the patient. Peripheral techniques used at the metacarpals, phalanges, wrist, tibia, and calcaneus include radiographic absorptiometry (RA), dual-energy X-ray absorptiometry (DXA), and quantitative ultrasound (QUS) and have made bone mass measurements more accessible and affordable. Dual-energy techniques, initially dual-energy photon absorptiometry (DPA), which now has been replaced by DXA, correct for soft tissue, obviating the need for water baths. Quantitated computerized tomography (QCT) assesses cancellous bone of the vertebral body and measures volumetric bone mineral density and bone size. Currently DXA of the axial skeleton, hip, and wrist offers the versatility of measuring multiple skeletal sites for the determination of bone mass and the proven ability to monitor the effects of drug therapy. Peripheral devices offer increased assessibility and affordability, fracture prediction, and diagnostic capabilities in the elderly. These measurements of bone mass have been statistically correlated with epidemiological and prospective fracture risk. This allows a clinician to estimate fracture risk for a patient based on bone mass measurements alone and diagnose low bone mass in appropriate populations.

Characteristics of bone vary in the axial and peripheral skeleton. The proportion of cortical to trabecular bone, metabolic activity, the effect of stress loading, and weight bearing all cause concern when trying to represent the entire skeleton by measurement at only one skeletal site or predict fracture at skeletal sites other than the one measured. This is particularly true in the early menopausal population, where bone mass is more discordant. Fracture of the hip or spine, because of their associated morbidity, mortality, and high financial burden, are the fractures for which fracture risk prediction is of most interest. Fracture risk is most accurately predicted by measurement of the specific bone for which it is desired, that is, measurement of femoral neck density most accurately predicts hip fracture risk. Yet global fracture prediction in the elderly can be determined by measuring bone mass at any skeletal site. The lower cost and increased availability of bone mineral density (BMD) measurements now allow more at-risk individuals to be tested, diagnosed, and treated.

BASIC PRINCIPLES OF DENSITOMETRY

Photon or X-ray attentuation by bone is directly proportional to ash weight density of bone. Ash weight, the residual after complete dehydration, represents mineral content and is proportionate to bone strength. Hence, bone mineral content is the most important determinant of the variance of bone strength and the resistance of bones to fracture. The accuracy of the densitometry method is determined by how closely the measurement of a cadaveric bone specimen matches its ash weight. The better the accuracy, the better a device measures the actual bone mineral content. Accuracy is largely dependent on the soft tissue surrounding the bone. Since less soft tissue surrounds the peripheral skeleton, the peripheral skeletal measurements are more accurate. The more accurate the device, the lower the diagnostic variability as defined by standard deviations. The precision of each technique is a description of the reproducibility of mutiple measurements of a single specimen. See Table 4-1.

The measurement accuracy for determining bone mineral content per unit volume of bone should not be confused with the accuracy of the technique to predict fracture. Precision, expressed as a percentage of the coefficient of variation (%CV), is important for determining significant change from one measurement to the next. The frequency of BMD scanning to determine the rate of BMD change is determined by the rate at which bone density at any given skeletal site is expected to change and the precision of the measurement technique at that site. The faster rate of change and more precise technique allow a shorter interval time for a statistically significant comparison between measurements.

CENTRAL MEASUREMENTS

Dual-Energy X-Ray Absorptiometry

Methods employing two energy peaks were developed to allow discrimination between soft tissue and bone. The low energy beam, partially attenuated by the soft tissue, allows quantification of soft tissue. The high energy beam is attenuated by both soft tissue and bone. Knowledge of soft tissue density provided by the low energy beam allows calculation of the fraction of the high energy beam attenuation attributable only to bone. From this fraction bone density is calculated. In practice central DXA is routinely performed at the lumbar spine and the proximal femur. Although there are close similarities between BMD measurement at one site versus another (Pearson's coefficient of variation ranging from 0.5 to 0.8), this similarity is not statistically strong enough to predict a BMD value at one site from another in individual patients.

The dual-energy technique allows for additional quantification measurements. Hip and spine scans are routinely performed in the PA projection, but later positioning allows for BMD determination in the lateral view, which removes the artifactual elevations of BMD that often occur in the elderly. Lateral BMD by DXA is highly correlated with axial QCT BMD, which also measures predominantly cancellous bone and is correlated to bone fragility. Lateral DXA scans also can be used for quantitative vertebral morphometry of the vertebrae for calculation of vertebral height and thus identification of partial vertebral collapse or progression of vertebral fracture. Periprosthetic loosening due to demineralization, the predominant cause for repeat hip replacement surgery, is not precisely, or with optimal sensitivity, identifiable on radiographs. The Gruen zones devised for the radiographic diagnosis of periprosthetic loosening may be applied to the DXA scan for region of interest quantification of periprosthetic bone mineral. The mechanics of the scanning table is designed for head to toe scanning, which allows measurement of total body calcium, for example, to measure increased bone mass during adolescent growth or as a result of therapy. This head to toe dual-energy scanning also allows analysis of body composition and the determination of lean and fat body mass.

Quantitated Computerized Tomography

Quantitated computerized tomography was adapted for bone densitometry in the 1970s. It offers the advantages of computerized tomography (CT), high resolution images, the ability to view vertebrae in the transverse plane, and segregation of cortical from trabecular bone. Density can be measured in its true parameters, grams per centimeter cubed, rather than the areal density, grams per centimeter squared, obtained from DXA measurements. Assessment of vertebral bone size by quantitating volumetric bone mass may have advantages over areal bone assessments since bone size becomes important in bone strength in certain populations, although to date the data do not suggest substantial fracture predictive capabilities by measuring areal bone mineral density, volumetric bone mineral density, or apparent bone mineral density, a derived DXA determination. Peripheral QCT of the wrist, a technology which employs a dedicated CT scanner to evalaute cortical and trabecular bone in the easily accessible distal forearm, is limited by its inability to discriminate between individuals with and without osteoporotic fracture.

Radiographic Absorptiometry and Single-Energy X-Ray Absorptiometry

Radiographic absorptiometry (RA) was developed in the 1960s and consists of a plain radiograph of the hand justaposed to an aluminum wedge with gradation of width calibrated to ash weight density. Distal radial single-energy X-ray absorptiometry (SXA) and DXA have an accuracy of about 94% and low precision error of 1–2%.

Quantitative Ultrasound

Ultrasound waves are attenuated, change in shape, intensity, and speed, when transmitted through tissue. Cancellous bone (the calcaneus is 95% cancellous) causes sound waves to scatter, whereas cortical bone absorbs them. Broadband ultrasound attenuation (BUA) measured in decibels (dB) is reduced in porous bone. The speed of sound (SOS) is calculated by measuring the width of the heel, divided by the time required for the sound to travel through the heel, and is decreased when bone density is less. The greatest effect on the wave is produced by bone mineral, but there is theoretically a component of bone quality, trabecular connectivity, which may also be represented. Calcaneal QUS parameters, BUA and SOS, linearly correlated with BMD, and the coefficient of variation (r value) relating BMD of the heel by DXA and ultrasound parameters is about 0.85. Several derived parameters of ultrasound (the stiffness index or the BMD) are composite indexes of both SOS and BUA. Both parameters are also highly correlated with heel DXA and/or AP spine DXA. Tibial ultrasound was also recently approved by the FDA, and tibial ultrasound SOS parameters have been associated with fracture risk prediction. Ultrasound is an attractive technique because it employs no ionizing radiation and the equipment is small, lightweight, and portable. If measurements are obtained in a setting that promotes appropriate interpretation and follow-up, using the guidelines as established by the International Society for Clinical Densitometry (ISCD), this technique may be very helpful for diagnosing and treating patients who otherwise would remain untreated.

Quality Assurance

As with any diagnostic technique, BMD testing may be limited by the accuracy and precision of the equipment, the method in which the test is performed, and the interpretation of the results. Each of the manufacturers provide quality assurance procedures for maintenance of the accuracy and precision of the scanners, usually determined by phantom scanning. The manufaturers' reported precision error, expressed by the coefficient of variation (CV) is usually 1% CV for the AP spine and 1.5% for total hip. However, the *in vivo* precision error must be determined by each densitometer site and may not be the same in patients with low bone mass. The predominant source of imprecision is with performance of the test by the technologist. Inconsistent patient positioning and inconsistent analysis by a technologist may lead to calculated changes in measurements of statistical significance. The potential for error is amplified when the scans are performed by multiple technologists who are not solely dedicated to the task. Precision will vary from device to device, from technologist to technologist, from scanning center to scanning center, and with the baseline level of BMD. Because longitudinal patient assessment necessitates knowledge of the precision, each scanning center should determine the precision of their own technique.

Bone mass quantification is a new and still evolving technology that requires a new knowledge base for the physician using the test to diagnose and monitor therapy of patients. Some manufacturers of equipment have training programs, which are typically attended by the technologist who will be most frquently using the equipment. These programs are valuable for basic performance training. Ideally it is preferable to have a dedicated technologist for the performance of these measurements. The ISCD was organized, in part, to provide both physician and technologist training in order to promote standardization of technique and clarification of appropriate reporting. It would behoove the referring physician to query the densitometry sites he/she employs as to whether the reporting physician and technologist are accredited by this society. The instruction and guidelines provided by the ISCD certification course should result in better understanding and performance of these procedures.

Physicians and Bone Density Application

Bone densitometry must be used by all the types of physicians who care for postmenopausal patients, or patients with specialized forms of osteoporosis. The only hope for doctors to detect low bone mass in the approximately 80 million postmenopausal population in the next 20 years is by primary care physicians and various specialists, both working hand in hand to increase access to BMD testing. The challenge is to also ensure competent interpretation of the computer printout reports, which currently are not yet standardized and will always need individual clinical considerations. The discovery of low bone mass in the appropriate population is as valuable a predictor of fracture as high cholesterol or high blood pressure are as predictors of their respective clinical outcomes of myocardial infarction and stroke. Though risk factor assessments have educational patient awareness value, this does not discount the importance of assessing other risk factors for fracture. In conjunction with BMD, risk factors add valuable information required for decisions related to which patients should be treated. Also, some risk factors can be modified to help reduce fracture risk. This is particularly true in the perimenopausal population, or in patients with secondary conditions associated with bone loss.

DIAGNOSIS OF OSTEOPOROSIS USING BONE DENSITOMETRY: THE WORLD HEALTH ORGANIZATION CRITERIA

In order for quantitative BMD values to be utilized for the purpose of diagnosiing osteoporosis, a paradigm shift in the definition of osteoporosis had to occur. Even though the new composite defintion of osteoporosis includes the terms BMD, systemic microarchitectural deterioration, and increased bone fragility, only BMD can be clinically measured by physicians at the current time. Prior to the previous consensus statement defining osteoporosis, a diagnosis of osteoporosis was made after a fragility fracture had already occurred. Now osteoporosis can be defined on the basis of a certain reduced level of BMD. This definition was implemented in 1991 by the Consensus Development Conference on Osteoporosis and was completed in 1994 by a highly regarded committee of the World Health Organization (WHO).

The major justification for changing the diagnostic criteria for osteoporosis from one of prevalent fragility fractures to one of low BMD is data establishing the higher risk of a second fracture once the first fracture has occurred. There is a far greater risk of additional vertebral fractures as well as hip fracture following the first vertebral fracture, or a second hip fracture after the first hip fracture. This risk is far greater than the increased risk of a first fracture in elderly individuals who have low bone mass alone.

The WHO criteria for the diagnosis of osteopenia and osteoporosis (Table 4-1) are based on a patient's comparison to peak adult bone mass

TABLE 4-1. World Health Organization Criteria for the Diagnosis of Osteopenia and Osteoporosis

Osteopenia = T-score < -1.0 and > -2.5
Osteoporosis = T-score < -2.5

(PABM) and use standardized scores (T-score). The WHO working group chose to categorize individuals using the number of standard deviations (SD) a patient's bone mass is below the mean of a young normal reference population bone mass. This removes the differences in actual BMD related to machine calibration observed using different manufacturers' equipment. The cutoff point of 2.5 SD below PABM is based on epidemiological data derived from a population of postmenopausal Caucasian women, more than 50% of whom had already suffered a fragility fracture of the hip, vertebra, wrist, humerus, or pelvis. The <-2.5 SD cutoff point was both prevalence-based and risk-based. The WHO working group recognized the arbitrary nature of the -2.5 SD level, because fracture risk is a gradient and not a threshold, and using prevalence data, the prevalence will increase as the number of skeletal sites are measured. Yet, since fracture risk is a gradient, increasing with declining levels of bone mass, the WHO created a second diagnostic category of osteopenia (low bone mass, T-score >-2.5 but <-1.0 SD) to alert the clinician that certain individuals with smaller reductions in bone mass may merit attention, particularly if they are postmenopausal, are not receiving estrogen replacement therapy, or have secondary conditions associated with potential bone loss.

Postmenopausal women who are not receiving hormonal replacement therapy (HRT) will predictably lose bone, as will most men and women receiving medications or diagnosed with medical conditions associated with bone loss. Since in the United States there are now three FDA approved agents for prevention, and since the recent National Osteoporosis Foundation (NOF) clinical guidelines recommend early prevention intervention (postmenopausal women with T-score >-1.5 SD with one or more risk factors), the diagnostic category of osteopenia may take on increasing importance as well. Hence, postmenopausal women identified as "osteopenic" may be targeted for prevention strategies to preserve their skeletal mass. Individuals with osteopenia may also experience fragility fractures, particularly when risk factors for fractures are present; untreated early postmenopausal women with low bone mass have an increased immediate risk of fracture. Such factors include increased risk of bone turnover, advancing age, and increased likelihood of falling.

As for all diagnostic criteria, there are strengths and limitations in the WHO criteria for the diagnosis of osteoporosis. These are listed in Table 4-2. The WHO criteria provide the busy practitioner with an objective number to be used for the diagnosis of osteoporosis, akin to a blood pressure level of 140/90 for the diagnosis of hypertension. Practitioners are now provided with objective criteria that initiate the cognitive process of assessment leading to intervention. In addition, the WHO criteria stresses the importance of making a diagnosis of low bone mass (osteopenia) or osteoporosis before the first fracture occurs.

The limitations presented in Table 4-2 appear to outnumber the strengths. However, this should not discount the beneficial impact that BMD measurements and the WHO criteria have had in the prevention and management

TABLE 4-2. World Health Organization Criteria for the Diagnosis of Osteopenia/Osteoporosis, Pros and Cons

Pro
1. Provides a simple objective diagnostic number for practitioners to use.
2. Recognizes that osteoporosis should be diagnosed prior to the first fragility fracture.

Con
1. Limited data relating WHO criteria to fracture risk in other races or genders.
2. Dependent on peak adult bone mass reference databases.
3. Not all low bone mass is osteoporosis.
4. Fracture risk is a gradient, not a threshold, and −2.5 SD may be used as a threshold cutoff.
5. Application to healthy premenopausal, estrogen-replete women and young men is inappropriate.

of osteoporosis. The WHO criteria have facilitated the widespread measurement of bone mass for the identification of individuals at risk for fracture.

One of the limitations of the WHO criteria is its limited applicability to women of other races and to men. The WHO <−2.5 SD cutoff criteria are recommended because this level captures the majority of prevalent fractures in postmenopausal Caucasian women and projections of lifetime fracture risk. Similar data in men and women of other racial groups are not well established. Some studies have suggested that fracture rates in elderly Caucasian men per standard deviation (SD) reduction in BMD nearly approximate that seen in Caucasian women, whereas others suggest the risk might be lower although still predictive. As prospective fracture data are obtained for other races, the applicability of the WHO criteria can accurately be judged as it relates to risk. BMD data for the hip were analyzed from the extensive National Health and Nutrition Examination Survey III (NHANES III), in men and women of different races. These data have helped determine the prevalence of osteoporosis at the hip in men and women of different races, using the WHO criteria. The incorporation of this common reference database into DXA equipment by the three major manufacturers has eliminated the potential for machine-specific misdiagnoses of osteoporosis or osteopenia at the hip. The T-scores are calculated from a common hip young normal reference database, rather than from manufacturer-specific hip databases.

Skeletal sites and bone density manufacturers for all other skeletal site measurements still use nonuniform (manufacturer-specific) reference databases. This is a critical issue in the field of bone densitometry. The T-score is calculated as follows:

$$T\text{-score} = \frac{(\text{Patient's BMD}) - (\text{Mean BMD of the young normal reference population})}{\text{SD of the BMD of the young normal reference population}}$$

As a consequence, an individual may be classiifed by *T*-scores quite differently even at the same skeletal site if different young normal reference populations are used to create the reference database to which the patient is compared. This presents serious clinical problems since a patient may be classified differently by various bone mass measurement devices when nonuniform young normal reference databases are used. Such a manufacturer-specific *T*-score, which classifies individuals differently, will lead to bone mass measurement credibility issues, and patient misclassification which has other implications to payers and the pharmaceutical industry. These issues could be resolved, in large part, by the creation of a standardized uniform young reference database for each skeletal site and technique, which could be adapted by all the major manufacturers. Validating this latter point are data showing that in postmenopausal women bone mass measured by various heel measuring devices (several ultrasound and heel DXA machines) and hip DXA have similar *T*-scores, when the *T*-score is calculated from the same young normal reference population. This finding supports the concept that differences in *T*-scores may be related more to different young normal reference populations than to technology or skeletal site differences.

A uniform BMD database could become the gold standard to which future databases would be compared as new techniques emerge. Presently, this uniform database does not exist; it is work in progress. The common "mother" young normal reference database will take approximately 2 years to complete, since it will also be validated by measuring elderly postmenopausal women, the "grandmother" set, both without and with prevalent fractures.

In the interim, a short-term solution to the *T*-score discrepancy is being developed by a committee of the NOF/ISCD in cooperation with equipment manufacturers. The development of the "*T*-score equivalence" is based on equal prevalence defined by all devices (equal to the 50% prevalence observed in NHANES III at the femoral neck in 60- to 69-year-old Caucasian women) (Figure 4-1). The −1.5 SD cutoff level was chosen because the *T*-score level of −1.5 SD is related to the equal global fracture prediction of all devices in elderly postmenopausal women, is related to the NOF's treatment threshold in postmenopausal women with one or more risk factors, and, for the femoral neck values, will capture >60% of the osteoporotic fractures in elderly Caucasian women. It may also evolve that *T*-score equivalence for all devices may also be expressed as equivalent fracture risk. This latter way of expressing equivalent *T*-scores between devices depends on the presence of adequate fracture data for all devices. It may not be necessary for manufacturers to obtain prospective fracture data, but cross-sectional fracture data, which tend to track well with prospective data, will be necessary to define equivalent risk. It may be necessary to express *T*-score equivalence as both prevalence and risk since clinicians still need a number (i.e., −2.5 SD) to make a diagnosis. Patients want to know if they have the "disease," and furthermore our reimbursement system requires specific diagnostic codes (ICD-9) for payment of services.

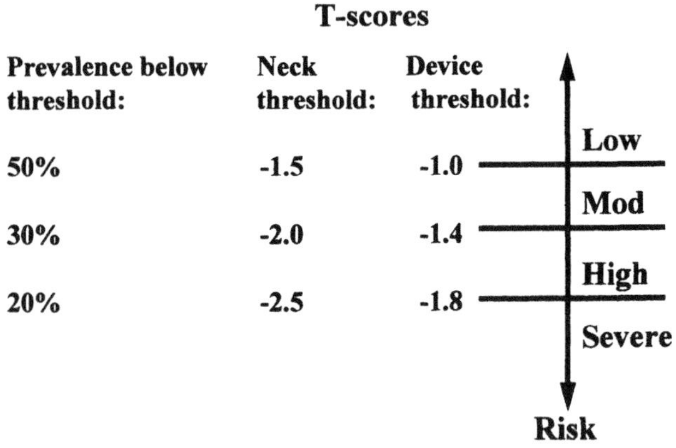

T-scores

Prevalence below threshold:	Neck threshold:	Device threshold:	
			Low
50%	-1.5	-1.0	
			Mod
30%	-2.0	-1.4	
			High
20%	-2.5	-1.8	
			Severe

Risk

Fig. 4-1. An example of how T-score equivalence can be used to equate the T-score from a specific bone mass measurement device to T-scores associated with the NHANES III femoral neck T-score. (Adapted from work performed by Black D, Miller P, Watts, Johnston C, Lindsay R, and Faulkner K.)

The lack of a standardized reference database notwithstanding, the various devices themselves measure bone mineral content per unit volume of bone with extraordinary accuracy and precision.

The WHO chose to define osteoporosis on the basis of the *T*-score, the comparison to the PABM rather than the *Z*-score, the comparison to age-matched bone mass. Although bone mass declines with advancing age, it is illogical to assume that bone loss is desirable or inevitable. If only those individuals who lose more bone than predicted for their age are termed "diseased," then many individuals with increased risk of fracture will go unrecognized and untreated. Therefore, even though the bone mass may be at a level that is expected for the age of the patient, the risk of fracture is increased, and it would be illogical to classify such a bone mass as "normal." If the prevalence of osteoporosis were defined using age-matched BMD data, it would not increase with age. This is an illogical approach since declining bone mass increases the risk for fracture and fracture is the outcome of the disease osteoporosis. Using age-matched *Z*-scores would result in the underdiagnosis of osteoporosis. This would damage the credibility of bone densitometry by the incorrect reporting "normal for age" in elderly patients with fragile skeletons or possibly even prevalent fragility fractures.

Even if 70% of Caucasian women over the age of 80 years have osteoporosis using the WHO criteria, this is not an overdiagnosis since 50% of these women will suffer a fragility fracture if left untreated. Using PABM as the diagnostic level for comparisons recognizes the true magnitude of the osteoporotic problem. Age-matched data are appropriate for comparisons in the growing child or adolescent; however, once PABM is achieved, the desirable clinical goal is to maintain the bone density at that level, not accept losses in excess of those predicted with age. It has been suggested that age-matched Z-scores which are less than -2.0 SD may indicate the presence of a metabolic process causing bone loss other than aging or estrogen deficiency in the postmenopausal population. Though intuitively correct, this suggestion remains an untested hypothesis.

The WHO criteria, as a diagnostic criteria, were never meant to be applied clinically to healthy, estrogen-replete premenopausal women. The inappropriate use of these diagnostic criteria may cause undue fear in premenopausal women regarding fracture risk and the initiation of inappropriate or excessive therapy. While some cross-sectional data suggest that healthy, estrogen-replete premenopausal women may slowly lose bone mass at the hip, other longitudinal data suggest that healthy, estrogen-replete premenopausal women may not be losing bone mass. In addition, healthy premenopausal women with low bone mass may not have any greater current fracture risk than their age-matched peers with normal BMD. The scant fracture data available in young people are either cross-sectional or have small numbers of patients with wide confidence intervals. Healthy young individuals may be inappropriately restricted in their activities or have reduced quality of life by the inappropriate applicaton of the WHO criteria intended to relate BMD to prevalent fractures in elderly populations. Since PABM follows a normal distribution, the discovery of low bone mass (even a T-score of -2.5 SD) in healthy premenopausal women does not necessarily mean that prior bone loss has occurred. It may simply represent a genetically or environmentally determined low PABM.

Healthy estrogen-replete premenopausal women should not receive BMD testing. However, such individauls who do obtain a BMD test and seek professional advice may require assessment to exclude secondary causes of potential bone loss, conservative prevention advice, a repeat bone mass measurement in 2 years to reassure them that bone loss is not occurring, and prompt protection of their skeleton at the menopause. There are presently no data to suggest that currently available pharmacological intervention with bisphosphonates, calcitonin, or estrogen analogs have any value in the premenopausal, estrogen-replete woman. These women may become pregnant, and the effect of these agents on fetal outcomes is unclear.

WHY ARE BONE MASS MEASUREMENTS PERFORMED?

There are three clinical applications for bone mass measurement. Each has a distinct value in clinical decision making. The three applciations are

1. Diagnosis of osteopenia or osteoporosis
2. Fracture risk prediction
3. Serial monitoring to measure response to intervention(s) or diseases/ medications that effect bone

TABLE 4-3. Techniques for Bone Mass Measurement

Central Skeleton
DXA—spine (AP or lateral), or hip
QCT—spine or hip
Peripheral Skeleton
DXA—wrist, heel, finger
QCT—wrist
Ultrasound—calcaneus, finger, tibia

The clinician has at their disposal various devices that measure bone mineral density. These devices are characterized as central or peripheral. Central devices measure the spine or the hip, and peripheral devices measure the wrist, heel, or finger. These devices are listed in Table 4-3. For each of the three applications of bone density measurement listed above, the central and peripheral devices have advantages and disadvantages.

1. The Diagnosis of Osteopenia and Osteoporosis

The diagnosis of osteopenia (T-score of <-1.0 but >-2.5) is clinically important independent of fracture risk assessment. This diagnostic category represents the range of bone density for which prevention strategies for early postmenopausal bone loss are designed. It has been shown that women who are made aware that their bone mass is low more readily accept hormone replacement therapy (HRT). It will most likely be the same for the other FDA-approved interventions for the prevention of early postmenopausal bone loss such as bisphosphonates and the selective estrogen receptor modulators (SERMs). These agents are recommended for the prevention of bone loss in postmenopausal women with T-scores <-1.5 who are unwilling or unable to utilize HRT.

The reliabiilty of central or peripheral sites in detecting osteopenia is dependent on the age of the patient and the particular skeletal site measured. BMD is discordant throughout the skeleton in addition to the discordance that is related to different young normal reference databases. This discordance is due, in part, to different accuracy errors of the different technologies, as well as different rates of age-related rates of bone loss from dissimilar BMD levels at PABM.

Because different rates of bone loss from different skeletal compartments begins at the menopause, discordance is greater (particularly between spine and hip) in the early menopausal population than in the elderly (>65 years) population. In the elderly, the greater concordance in BMD at various skeletal sites reduces the likelihood of missing a diagnosis of osteopenia or osteoporosis when only one skeletal site is measured. However, in the elderly, if only the AP spine is measured by DXA, osteophytes and/or facet sclerosis of the posterior elements may falsely increase the value causing misdiagnosis. In the elderly, central measurements except the AP spine and all peripheral measurements have equivalent value for diagnosing osteopenia or osteoporosis. Although central and peripheral BMD sites appear to have equal diagnostic utility in elderly women, this may not be true for perimenopausal women due to the greater skeletal discordance in BMD in this age group.

The degree of discordance is also T-score cutoff point dependent. For example, data suggest that in early menopausal women if one skeletal site is osteoporotic (T-score <-2.5 SD) then there is less than a 10% chance that any other skeletal site will be normal. Published studies have not yet clarified how many early postmenopausal women have normal BMD at one site and osteopenia (T-score -1.0 to -2.5 SD) at another. These numbers may not be insignificant. Hence, many early menopausal women may need additional BMD testing if a single skeletal site measurement, incrasingly being done with peripheral technology, is normal in order not to miss a diagnosis of osteopenia. This is particularly true if the woman has additional risk factors for low BMD or if a diagnosis of osteopenia would change the pharmacological preventive intervention. Patients with a normal single skeletal site BMD who may need additional BMD tests are described in Table 4-4. These guidelines are required to minimize the potential for misdiagnosis.

There are other patient populations in which a diagnosis of osteopenia may lead to changes in intervention strategies. The prevention of bone loss associated with glucocorticoid therapy is recommended in patients with T-scores below -1.0. It may also be appropriate to intervene in other medical conditions associated with bone loss (hyperthyroidism, hyperparathyroidism, posttransplantation, etc.) based on a finding of osteopenia.

2. The Prediction of Fracture Risk

There is little debate that low bone mass is the most important predictor of fragility fracture. Approximately 80% of the variance in bone strength and resistance of bone to fracture in animal models is explained by the bone

TABLE 4-4. Patients with a Normal Peripheral Bone Mass Who May Need Additional Bone Mass Testing

1. Postmenopausal patients concerned about osteoporosis, not receiving HRT, but would accept HRT, bisphosphonates, or SERMs if BMD is found to be low.
2. Patients at high risk for hip fracture, who have a maternal history of hip fracture, who are $>5'7''$ tall, who weigh >127 lb., or who smoke.
3. Patients receiving medications associated with bone loss (e.g., glucocorticoids, antiseizure medications, chronic heparin).
4. Patients with secondary conditions associated with low bone mass or bone loss (e.g., hyperparathyroidism, malabsorption, hemigastrectomy, hyperthyroidism).
5. Patients found to have high urinary collagen cross-links (>1.0 SD above the upper limit for premenopausal women), where more rapid bone loss may be present.
6. Patients with a history of fragility fractures.

mineral content per unit volume of bone. Other risk factors are predictive of fracture; however, some are not as objectively quantifiable as bone mass and some are not modifiable. Risk factors such as increased height (>5'7"), low body weight (<127 lb.), smoking, or maternal history of hip fracture are strong predictors of hip fracture. However, BMD is an objective, quantifiable measurement that offers clinical value akin to showing a patient their blood pressure or cholesterol measurement on a printed sheet. Bone loss can now be halted and gains in bone density can be achieved. Increased height or maternal history of hip fracture independently increase fracture risk, but there is no way to modify these risk factors.

The relationship between fracture risk and bone density is best described as a gradient rather than a threshold, and this gradient becomes more than exponential at T-scores <−2.5 SD (Fig. 4-2). Fracture prediction can be expressed as current fracture risk or lifetime fracture risk. Current risk is the risk of fracture within 3–5 years after the measurement of bone mass and has been established in prospective studies in elderly postmenopausal women and elderly men. Current fracture risk can be expressed as relative risk (RR), absolute risk of incidence, or annual risk. Relative risk, the ratio of two ab-

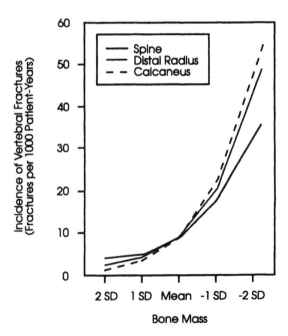

Fig. 4-2. Exponential relationship between decreasing bone mass and increasing incidence of vertebral fractures. (Reprinted by permission of the Society of Nuclear Medicine from: Wasnich RD, et al. A comparison of single and multi-site BMC measurements for assessment of spine fracture probability. *Journal of Nuclear Medicine*. 1989; 30:1166–1171.)

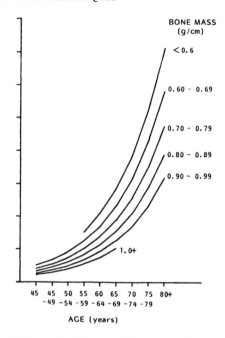

BONE MASS
(g/cm)

< 0.6

0.60 - 0.69

0.70 - 0.79

0.80 - 0.89

0.90 - 0.99

1.0+

45   45   50   55   60   65   70   75   80+
     -49 -54 -59 -64 -69 -74 -79

AGE (years)

Fig. 4-3. Estimated incidence of facture as a function of age.

solute risks, is increased 1.5–3 times for each 1.0 SD reduction in BMD. In addition, fracture risk is greater as age increases at the same level of BMD, particularly in patients above age 65 (Figure 4-3). This greater fracture risk at the same level of BMD is due to age-related alterations in bone quality which is not clinically measurable.

Since bone loss is an asymptomatic process, identifying small reductions in bone mass in early menopausal patients is important to allow early intervention to halt bone loss, since fracture risk will continue to increase as BMD decreases and age increases. Some patients will fracture with BMD which is only minimally reduced (osteopenia) due to the effects of other factors that lead to bone fragility. In some of these patients, the rate of bone turnover or the nature of a fall may lead to fracture with only minimal reduction in BMD.

All the current fracture risk data available in the elderly suggest that fracture prediction is not dependent on the skeletal site measured or the technique (central or peripheral) used. This observation is probably related to the greater concordance of bone mass at different skeletal sites in the elderly population. Thus, in this elderly population, low BMD measured at one site is more likely to represent a global reduction in BMD. The only exception is the prediction of hip fracture risk, which appears to be better if the BMD at the proximal femoral sites are used. This observation does not, however, diminish the strong predictive value that peripheral bone mass measurement has for the prediction of hip fracture. Data on current fracture risk have been obtained only in elderly Caucasian women due to the fact that younger women fracture infrequently and are not, therefore, included in studies designed to determine current fracture risk. Because of the powerful independent effect of increasing age on fracture risk, the current fracture risk is much lower in the 50-year-old woman versus the 75-year-old woman at comparable BMD levels.

Lifetime fracture risk models, however, have value in counseling this elderly menopausal population. The 50-year-old woman with low BMD and no treatment to prevent bone loss may have a greaer lifetime fracture risk than her 50-year-old counterpart with a normal BMD because she is starting the menopause with a lower bone mass.

Most postmenopausal women lose bone mass after the menopause without intervention. Therefore, untreated postmenopausal women expected to lose bone mass as they age will progressively have a lower BMD as they age. All lifetime fracture prediction models are hypothetical, and they have not yet been (nor probably ever will be) validated by direct longitudinal data. Clinically, however, it is useful to discuss the implications of low bone mass at the menopause relative to probable lifetime fracture risk, since it may facilitate the acceptance of HRT or other pharmacological prevention interventions early in the menopause.

3. Serial Assessments of Bone Mass

Bone densitometry can be used for serial monitoring of the natural progression of disease processes (such as primary hyperparathyroidism) or for monitoring the response of bone to pharmacological interventions. There is currently a clear advantage of the central skeleton over the peripheral skeleton for serial monitoring. In monitoring the response of bone to estrogens, SERMs, bisphosphonates, or calcitonin, the axial skeleton consistently demonstrates the greatest magnitude of change in the shortest time. The femur tends to demonstrate changes in rsponse to pharmacological interventions, though at rates lower than the spine, while little or no change is observed at the wrist, finger, or heel. The reason peripheral skeletal sites have a limited BMD measurable rsponse to pharmacological intervention is unclear. It is not due to the precision of the measurement of peripheral techniques, which is excellent (1.0%). Several hypotheses have been suggested to explain this observation, such as differences in the bone marrow environment of the peripheral skeleton versus the central skeleton, differences in surface area of bone, and differences in blood flow between the two bone compartments. No matter which hypothesis is correct, the reality is that the response of BMD to treatment is more readily detectable at the spine and hip. There are some limited data suggesting that forearm bone mass measurements may be useful in monitoring the response to HRT in individual patients and that calcaneal ultrasound may show changes to pharmacological interventions as well. These studies need to be repeated and confirmed.

The forearm appears to be the best skeletal site to monitor the effects of excess parathyroid hormone activity. It may also be valuable in decisions regarding the timing of surgical parathyroidectomy.

The change observed between serial BMD measurements can be expressed as percent change (% change) between two measurements or absolute change (in g/cm^2) between two measurements. Percent change is calculated as

$$\frac{\text{1st BMD} - \text{2nd BMD}}{\text{1st BMD}} \times 100 = \% \text{ Change}$$

Absolute change is calculated as

$$\text{1st BMD} - \text{2nd BMD} = \text{Absolute Change}$$

Change expressed in either format is acceptable, providing the precision of the measurement is available from the testing facility.

Individual DXA manufacturers may publish precision errors of 1% or less at the AP spine when, in fact, their precision error may be 3–4% in the elderly population with low BMD values (Fig. 4-4). This is due to an increased precision error (coefficient of variation) as the BMD declines at each skeletal site. In addition, variability may be introduced by the technologist during positioning or analysis, which will increase the precision error even in individuals with normal BMD. Once the precision error is known, then the significance of a change in serial BMD may be determined. At the 95% confidence level, a significant percent change in two serial BMD values is at least 2.77 times the known precision error. For example, if the precision error is 1.5%, then a 4.16% change (magnitude of change necessary for 95% confidence = 1.5% × 2.77 or 4.16%) is required between two BMD measurements to be signficant at the 95% confidence level. However, if the precision error is 3%, then it would require almost a 9% change (magnitude of

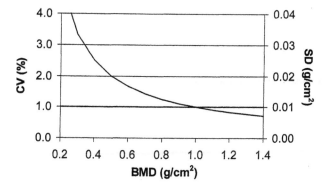

Fig. 4-4. As bone mineral density (BMD) decreases, the precision error (CV%) of the measurement increases (Faulkner K, unpublished data).

change necessary for 95% confidence = 3% × 2.77 or 8.31%) to be 95% confident that a true change in BMD has occurred. Misleading conclusions may be drawn, based on nonsignificant serial changes, with attending inappropriate alterations in treatments, if a densitometry facility precision errors are not known.

In contrast, absolute change in serial BMD is not nearly as influenced by precision error differences because the SD of BMD is reasonably constant over a wide range of BMD. Any absolute change in BMD greater than 0.04 g/cm^2 at the AP spine or 0.05 g/cm^2 at the femoral neck will generally be significant at the 95% confidence level. By convention in the medical literature, serial change has generally been expressed as a percentage; however, either method described above is valid.

Bone mineral density testing for serial monitoring is generally performed no more often than every 12–24 months, depending on the disease process or therapeutic intervention being monitored. In patients who have a documented response to pharmacological intervention, which may be defined as either a gain or no loss in BMD, annual BMD measurements may not be necessary. In patients with a documented response to HRT, repeat BMD measurements every 3–5 years may improve the poor long-term compliance to therapy. Even in elderly women who have been previously documented to be estrogen responders, a 3- to 5-year BMD testing interval may be used to document continued response and compliance to therapy, since age-related bone loss may induce BMD loss even with continual estrogen use.

It is very difficult to compare serial changes in BMD when the measurements are performed on different manufacturers' machines. It is often difficult to compare values obtained from different machines from the same manufacturer. It would be ideal if patients had serial measurements performed on the same machine by the same technician. However, this is unrealistic in today's world. Given the proprietary design of the various devices and the differences in calibration, the absolute BMD values from different machines in an individual patient will not be the same. Even when the machines are made by the same manufacturer, slight differences in calibration or differences in technique during data acquisition will introduce error. The establishment of the standardized BMD (sBMD), by the International Bone Densitometry Standards Committee, allows for better comparisons to be made between BMD values obtained on different manufacturers' equipment. Utilizing the calculated sBMD of the spine and hip for serial comparison reduces, but does not eliminate, the variance in the measurements. As a general rule, even when using sBMD, an additional 1% precision error should be added to the calculation of percent change.

CONCLUSIONS

Bone densitometry has revolutionized the clinical approach to osteoporosis. Much as the sphygmomanometer changed the field of hypertension and the prediction of the risk of stroke, bone densitometry provides a direct measurement of bone mineral density which is directly related to fracture risk. If the results of bone densitometry are used responsibly and competently, patient care will be enhanced. The measurement of bone mineral density enables physicians and their patients to make informed decisions regarding preventive and therapeutic strategies. It also allows the physician to monitor the longitudinal efficacy of these interventions.

SUGGESTED READING

Ahmed AIH, Blake GM, Rymer JM, Fogelman I: Screening for osteopenia and osteoporosis: Do the accepted normal ranges lead to overdiagnosis? Osteoporosis Int 7:432–438, 1997.

Arlot ME, Sornay-Rendu E, Garnero P, Vey-Marty B, Delmas PD: Apparent pre- and postmenopausal bone loss evaluated by DXA at different skeletal sites in women: The OLEFY cohort. J Bone Miner Res 12:683–690, 1997.

Baran DT, Faulkner KG, Genant HK, Miller PD, Pacifici R: Diagnosis and management of osteoporosis: Guidelines for the utilization of bone densitometry. Calcif Tissue Int 61:433–440, 1997.

Black DM, et al: Axial and appendicular bone density predict fractures in older women. J Bone Miner Res 7:633–638, 1992.

Black DM, Cummings SR, Melton LJ III: Appendicular bone mineral and a woman's lifetime risk of hip fracture. J Bone Miner Res 7:639–645, 1992.

Bonnick SL, Nichols DL, Sanborn CF, Lloyd K, Payne SG, Lewis L, Reed CA: Dissimilar spine and femoral Z-scores in premenopausal women. Calcif Tissue Int 61: 263–265, 1997.

Cauley JA, Seeley DG, Ensrud K, Ettinger B, Black D, Cummings SR. Estrogen replacement therapy and fracure in older women. Ann Intern Med 122:9–16, 1995.

Christiansen C, Lindsay R: Estrogens, bone loss and preservation. Osteoporosis Int 1:7–12, 1990.

Cummings SR: Treatable and untreatable risk factors for hip fracture. Bone 18:165S–167S, 1996.

Cummings SR, Black DM, Rubin SM: Lifetime risks of hip, Colles' or vertebral fracture and coronary heart disease among White postmenopausal women. Arch Intern Med 149:2556–2448, 1989.

Cummings, SR, Black DM, Nevitt MC, et al: Bone density at various sites for prediction of hip fracture. Lancet 341:72–75, 1993.

Cummings Sr, Nevitt MC, Browner WS, et al: Risk factors for hip fracture in White women. N Engl J Med 332:767–773, 1995.

Duppe H, Gardsell P, Nilsson B, Johnell O: A single bone density measurement can predict fractures over 25 years. Calcif Tissue Int 60:171–174, 1997.

Faulkner KG, McClung MR: Quality control of DXA instruments in multicenter trials. Osteoporosis Int 5:218–227, 1995.

Faulkner KG, Roberts LA, McClung MR: Discrepancies in normative data between Lunar and Hologic DXA system. Osteoporosis Int 6:432–436, 1996.

Finkelstein JS, Cleary RL, Butler JP, Antonelli R, Mitlak BH, Deraska DJ, Zamora-Quezada JC, Neer RM: A comparison of lateral versus anterior–posterior spine dual energy X-ray absorptiometry for the diagnosis of osteopenia. J. Clin Endocrinol Metab 78:724–730, 1994.

Garnero P, Hausherr E, Chapuy MC, et al: Markers of bone resorption predict hip fracture in elderly women: The EPIDOS prospective study. J Bone Miner Res 11:1531–1537, 1996.

Genant HK, Engelke K, Furst T, Gluer CC, Grampp S, Harris ST, Jergas M, Lang T, Lu V, Majumdar S, Mathur A, Takeda M: Noninvasive assessment of bone mineral and structure: State of the art. J Bone Miner Res 11:707–730, 1996.

Goulding A, Cannan R, Williams SM, Gold EJ, Taylor RW, Lewis-Barned NJ: Bone mineral density in girls with forearm fractures. J Bone Miner Res 13:143–148, 1998.

Grampp S, Genant HK, Mathur A, Lang P, Jergas M, Takada M, Gluer CC, Lu Y, Chavez M: Comparisons of noninvasive bone mineral measurements in assessing age-related loss, fracture discrimination, and diagnostic classification. J Bone Miner Res 12:697–711, 1997.

Greenspan SL, Myers ER, Maitland LA, Resnick NM, Hayes WC: Fall severity and bone mineral density as risk factors for hip fracture in ambulatory elderly. JAMA 271:128–133, 1994.

Greenspan SL, Maitland-Ramsey L, Myers E: Classification of osteoporosis in the elderly is dependent on site-specific analysis. Calcif Tissue Int 58:409–414, 1995.

Greenspan SL, Bouxein ML, Melton ME, Kolodny AH, Clair JH, Delucca PT, Stek M Jr, Faulkner KG, Orwoll ES: Precision and discriminatory ability of calcaneal bone assessment technologies. J Bone Miner Res 12:1303–1313, 1997.

Hans D, Dargent-Molina P, Scott AM, et al: Ultrasonographic heel measurements to predict hip fracture in elderly women: The EPIDOS prospective study. Lancet 348:511–514, 1996.

Hans D, Duboeuf F, Schott AM, Horn S, Avioli LV, Drezner MK, Meunier PJ: Effects of a new positioner on the precision of hip bone mineral density measurements. J Bone Miner Res 12:1289–1294, 1997.

Heilmann P, Wuster C, Prolingheuer C, Gotz M, Ziegler R: Measurement of forearm bone mineral density: Comparison of precision of five different instruments. Calcif Tissue Int 62:383–387, 1998.

Huang C, Ross PD, Wasnich RD: Short-term and long-term fracture prediction by bone mass measurements: A prospective study. J Bone Miner Res 13:107–113, 1998.

Hui SL, Slemenda CW, Johnston CC Jr: Age and bone mass as predictors of fracture in a prospective study. J Clin Invest 81:1804–1809, 1988.

Jergas M, Genant HK: Current methods and recent advances in the diagnosis of osteoporosis. Arth Rheum 36:1649–1662, 1993.

Kanis JA: Diagnosis of osteoporosis. Osteoporosis Int 7(S3):S108–S116, 1997.

Looker AC, Wahner HW, Dunn WL, et al: Proximal femur bone mineral levels of US adults. Osteoporosis Int 5:389–409, 1995.

Lufkin EG, Wahner HW, O'Fallon WM, Hodgson SF, Kotowicz MA, Lane AW, Judd HL, Caplan RH, Riggs BL: Treatment of postmenopausal osteoporosis with transdermal estrogen. Ann Intern Med 117:1–9, 1992.

Lunt M, Felsenberg D, Reeve J, et al: Bone density variation and its effect on risk of vertebral deformity in men and women studied in thirteen European centers: The EVOS study. J Bone Miner Res 12:1883–1894, 1997.

Marshall D, Johnell O, Wedel H: Meta-analysis of how well measures of bone mineral density predict occurrence of osteoporotic fractures. Br Med J 312:1254–1259, 1996.

Miller PD, McCluing M: Prediction of fracture risk I: Bone density. Am J Med Sci 312:257–259, 1996.

Miller PD, Bonnick SL, Rosen CJ, Altman RD, Avioli LV, Dequeker J, Felsenberg D, Genant HK, Gennari C, Harper KD, Hodsman AB, Kleerekoper M, Mautalen CA, McClung MR, Meunier PJ, Nelson DA, Peel NFA, Raisz LG, Recker RR, Utian WH, Wasnich RD, Watts NB: Clinical utility of bone mass measurements in adults: Consensus of international panel. Semin Arth Rheum 25:361–372, 1996.

Miller PD, Bonnick SL, Johnston CC Jr, Kleerekoper M, Lindsay RL, Sherwood LM, Siris ES: The challenges of peripheral bone density testing. *J. Clin Densitometry* 1:1–7, 1998.

Musolino ME, Looker AC, Madans JH, Langlois JA, Orwoll ES: Risk factors for hip fracture in White men: The NHANES I epidemiological follow-up study. J Bone Miner Res 13:918–925, 1998.

Nelson DA, Molloy R, Kleerekoper M: Prevalence of osteoporosis in women referred for bone density testing: Utility of multiple skeletal sites. J Clin Densitometry 1:5–12, 1998.

Pouilles JM, Ribot C, Tremollieres F, *et al:* Risk factors of vertebral osteoporosis: Results of a study of 2279 women referred to a menopause clinic. Rev Rheum Mal Osteoartc 58:169–177, 1991.

Pouilles JM, Tremollieres F, Ribot C: Spine and femur densitometry at the menopause: Are both sites necessary in the assessment of the risk of osteoporosis? Calcif Tissue Int 52:344–347, 1993.

Reid I: Glucocorticoid-induced osteoporosis: Assessment and treatment. J Clin Densitometry 1:55–65, 1998.

Riis BJ: Premenopausal bone loss: Fact or artifact? Osteoporosis Int S1:S35–S37, 1994.

Riis BJ, Hansen MA, Jensen AM, Overgaard K, Christiansen C: Low bone mass and fast rate of bone loss at menopause: Equal risk factors for future fracture: A 15-year follow-up study. Bone 19:9–12, 1996.

Ross PD, Davis JW, Epstein RS, Wasnich RD: Pre-existing fractures and bone mass predict vertebral fracture incidence in women. Ann Intern Med 114:919–923, 1991.

Rubin SM, Cummings SR: Results of bone densitometry affect women's decisions about taking measures to prevent fractures. Ann Intern Med 116:990–995, 1992.

Silverberg SJ, Shane E, de la Cruz L, *et al:* Skeletal disease in primary hyperparathyroidism. J Bone Miner Res 4:283–291, 1989.

The WHO Study Group: Assessment of Fracture Risk and Its Application to Screening for Postmenopausal Osteoporosis. Geneva: World Health Organization, 1994.

Watts NB, Harris ST, Genant HK, *et al:* Intermittent cyclic etidronate treatment of postmenopausal osteoporosis. N Engl J Med 323:73–79, 1990.

Yates AJ, Ross PD, Lydick E, Epstein RS: Radiographic absorptiometry in the diagnosis of osteoporosis. Am J Med 8(S2A):41S–47S, 1995.

5 Biochemical Markers of Bone Turnover

Roberto Civitelli

INTRODUCTION

Bone mass is the result of a lifelong balance between the processes of bone formation and resorption. In the adult skeleton, bone remodeling (turnover) is the fundamental physiologic mechanism that allows repair of injuries, such as fractures, renewal of aging bone tissue, and rearrangement of the skeletal architecture to maximize its flexibility to stress and resistance to load. Most metabolic bone diseases, including osteoporosis are the consequence of an unbalanced bone remodeling. Osteoporotic syndromes are characterized by a wide spectrum of bone turnover, ranging from accelerated to reduced remodeling rates. Although the status of bone remodeling is not pathognomonic of any particular condition, assessment of bone turnover rates adds information that may be helpful for estimating the severity of the condition and for selecting the most appropriate therapeutical approach. Recent work also indicates that bone turnover rate may be a good predictor of risk for fractures in osteoporosis.

Bone turnover can be precisely assessed by bone histomorphometry (see Chapter 13 in this volume). However, bone biopsy is not part of the routine evaluation of the osteoporotic patient because it is an invasive procedure that requires specialized laboratories and personnel for processing and evaluation. In analogy, calcium kinetics and balance studies, also used to assess bone turnover require administration of radioactive material and long periods of observation, an unsuitable approach for a typical outpatient clinical setting. More available to the general practitioner, as well as to the specialty physician who manages osteoporotic patients, are some biochemical indices

TABLE 5-1. Biochemical Markers of Bone Turnover

Markers of Bone Formation
  Serum alkaline phosphatase
  Serum osteocalcin (BGP)
  Serum type I collagen propeptides
    C-terminal propeptide (PICP)
    N-terminal propeptide (PINP)
Markers of Bone Resorption
  Urine hydroxyproline
  Pyridinoline cross-links
    Free pyridinoline (Pyr) and deoxypyridinoline (D-Pyr)
    Urine N-terminal-to-helix cross-links (NTX)
    Urine C-terminal-to-helix cross-links (CTX)
    Serum C-terminal-to-helix cross-links (ICTP)
  Other less used bone resorption markers
    Serum tartrate-resistant acid phosphatase
    Urine hydroxylysine glycosides

---

that reflect the ongoing bone remodeling process. These biochemical markers are based on the measurement of blood or urine levels of either enzymatic activities produced by bone cells, or bone matrix components which pass into the circulation during bone apposition or resorption.

Biochemical markers of bone turnover with established or promising clinical relevance are listed in Table 5-1. Although such classification implies that each parameter is an indicator of either formation or resorption, this implication should not be assumed very strictly. In most metabolic bone diseases, and in particular osteoporosis bone formation and resorption are coupled, that is both processes are either increased, decreased, or normal. This explains why it is extremely difficult to establish, on a clinical basis, whether one biochemical marker is indeed a pure indicator of one particular phase of bone remodeling. In addition, matrix products can be released into the circulation during their synthesis (bone formation) and breakdown (bone resorption). Thus, in most cases each biochemical marker has to be considered as being prevalently associated with either bone formation or resorption.

Although bone turnover markers are potentially powerful clinical tools, the clinician should bear in mind some important considerations in interpreting the results of these tests in clinical practice. First of all, biochemical markers cannot discriminate whether changes in remodeling rates are the result of focal bone diseases or systemic conditions. In other words, an increased biochemical marker may reflect bone remodeling in the whole skeleton or represent a systemic dilution of the marker produced at extremely high rates by focal disorders (e.g., Paget's disease of bone, metastatic tumors). By the same token, because bone histomorphometry provides information on a limited area of bone tissue, it may not necessarily be representative of the entire skeleton. Consequently, finding bad correlations between biochemical and histomorphometric parameters of bone remodeling does not necessarily imply a failure of a certain index to predict a certain phase of bone remodeling, it may only reflect a sampling bias. It is also important to consider that the unequal specificity, sensitivity, and normality ranges of each marker preclude any quantitative comparison between formation and resorption rates. Finally, circulating levels of these markers can be influenced by factors other than bone turnover, such as liver uptake and metabolism, renal excretion, or uptake by osteoblasts. Therefore, careful clinical correlations are required for a correct interpretation of these tests.

PARAMETERS OF BONE FORMATION

Serum Alkaline Phosphatase

Alkaline phosphatase is a set of enzymes which hydrolyze a phosphoric ester bond from organic and inorganic substrates at an alkaline pH optimum. Three different genes encode for different tissue-specific isoenzymes, placental, intestinal and a so called bone-liver-kidney isoform, which undergoes posttranslational modifications, mainly on the carbohydrate side chains of the glycoprotein complex. This metabolic step confers "secondary" tissue specificity, and accounts for the different heat sensitivities and electrophoretic properties of the isoforms that are exploited for their identification.

Total alkaline phosphatase activity is measured in plasma or serum using a colorimetric assay, based on the property of the enzyme to hydrolyze the substrate *para*-nitrophenylphosphate, at 37°C. In normal individuals, total enzyme activity is mostly contributed to by the liver and bone isoforms, while the intestinal isoenzyme is present only in minimal amounts that raise after eating. The simplest and most widely used method of separation between the two major circulating moieties of alkaline phosphatase is heat inactivation based on the higher heat-lability at 56°C of the bone isoform, compared to the liver species. A residual activity of <20% after 10-min incubation at 56°C suggests that the specimen originally contained predominantly bone alkaline phosphatase. However, the sensitivity of this method is poor and quantitation is virtually impossible because of the strict dependence on substrate concentration, and pH, temperature, and protein content of the serum. In order to obtain a more precise assessment of the two isoforms, immunoassays based on antibodies specific for the bone isoenzyme have been successfully used in bone-specific alkaline phosphatase assays. Cross-reactivity with the liver isoenzyme is usually low, because of the much greater affinity of the antibodies for the circulating bone isoform. These assays can now be reliably used for precise estimation of a bone origin of high total alkaline phosphatase. Unlike osteocalcin (see below), bone-specific alkaline phosphatase is unaffected by glomerular filtration rate, a useful feature in patients with impaired renal function.

Following a pattern that is common to all the other biochemical markers, circulating alkaline phosphatase changes with age and menopause. In actively growing children, the enzyme activity is 2- to 3-fold higher than in adults, and it is believed to represent an increase of the bone isoform. Although both total and bone-specific alkaline phosphatase increases linearly with age in both men and women, menopause results in a sharp increase in women, an effect that is more evident with bone-specific assays than with total enzyme activity. The assumption that alkaline phosphatase activity reflects mainly bone formation rather than resorption is based on the fact that the enzyme is expressed as a constitutive protein by osteoblasts, the bone-forming cells. Indeed, clinical studies have demonstrated a significant, albeit weak correlation of the enzyme activity with kinetic and histologic parameters of bone formation, but only in diseases characterized by extremely elevated bone turnover, such as Paget's disease of bone and primary hyperparathyroidism. Unfortunately, most of the studies on postmenopausal osteoporotic women have failed to demonstrate such clear correlations, probably because of the poor sensitivity of the assay, and the relatively narrow range of bone turnover rates associated with this disease. Accordingly, higher levels of alkaline phosphatase have been reported in women with osteoporosis compared to normal individuals, but such differences are modest relative to the normal range and variability of the assay. Thus, alkaline phosphatase is a good indicator of bone turnover in Paget's disease of bone, but it is a poor diagnostic tool for the osteoporotic patient.

In patients with osteoporosis, total alkaline phosphatase increases during fracture healing. The raise in the circulating enzyme activity is detectable only after 7–10 days from the acute episode, and the levels usually return toward normal within 4–6 weeks, depending on the age of the patient and the presence of other underling conditions. Other pathologic conditions to be considered when interpreting an elevated alkaline phosphatase in an otherwise asymptomatic patient are primary hyperparathyroidism and Paget's disease of bone. In both cases the enzyme activity correlates with the extent of bone involvement, and it is almost exclusively accounted for by the bone isoform. More subtle increases in alkaline phosphatase may occur in conditions leading to a mineralization defect, such as vitamin D deficiency, aluminum intoxication, X-linked hypophosphatemic rickets, and hyperthyroidism, as well as following pulmonary embolization and myocardial infarction. Alkaline phosphatase can also be elevated in patients treated with gold salts, nonsteroidal anti-inflammatory agents, allopurinol, and oral hypoglycemic agents.

Serum Osteocalcin (Bone Gla-Protein)

Osteocalcin, also referred to as bone-Gla-protein (BGP), is a noncollagenous protein almost exclusively present in bone and dentin. Mature osteocalcin is a single chain, 49-amino acid peptide with three γ-carboxyglutamic acid (Gla) residues derived by posttranslational carboxylation of glutamic acid in the polypeptide chain. The Gla residues confer the molecule a very high affinity to calcium ions and hydroxyapatite. This process is vitamin-K dependent, analogous to the γ-carboxylation of some clotting factors containing Gla residues, with which osteocalcin shares structural homology. As such, γ-carboxylation is sensitive to warfarin, although the synthesis of the protein is not. Whereas prolonged treatment with warfarin does not appear to significantly impair bone formation in adults, exposure of the fetus to sodium warfarin during the first trimester may result in infants born with a hypoplastic saddle nose, punctuate calcifications in distal phalanges and vertebrae, and stubby fingers. The recent development of mice genetically deficient in BGP have demonstrated that this protein functions as an inhibitor of calcification, which is consistent with its production only at later stages of bone mineralization.

Of the total osteocalcin synthesized by bone cells, about 10–25% escapes into the circulation, where it can be measured by radioimmunoassays, and it is almost entirely cleared by glomerular filtration. Therefore, when renal function is severely impaired, circulating BGP increases dramatically commensurate with serum creatinine. Fragments of osteocalcin are removed from the bone by osteoclasts during the resorptive process. Although these cleavage products can pass into the blood stream, they are small peptides that in most cases do not bind to the antibodies employed for osteocalcin measurement. Thus, the contribution of bone resorption to total osteocalcin is believed to be modest. Serum BGP is a valid marker of bone turnover when resorption and formation are coupled, that is, postmenopausal osteoporosis, primary hyperparathyroidism, hyperthyroidism, and chronic renal failure. When the two remodeling phases are uncoupled, such as in multiple myeloma, chronic use of corticosteroids, or tumor associated hypercalcemia serum BGP correlates closely with bone formation. Therefore, BGP provides a reliable, specific index of bone formation. This notion is confirmed by the high correlation between osteocalcin and both static and dynamic indices of bone formation consistently observed on histomorphometry and calcium kinetic studies.

Osteocalcin is measured in serum or plasma by radioimmunoassays, based on antibodies raised against the bovine protein, which cross-react with the human molecule. Of the circulating osteocalcin, a fraction (5–20%) is present in undercarboxylated forms, which cannot bind to hydroxyapatite. A circadian rhythm is evident in both men and women, with 15% variation between peak at 4 A.M., and nadir usually occurring around 5 P.M. Likewise, serum osteocalcin increases during the luteal phase, reaching a peak at the end of the cycle. At this time, its levels are on average 20% higher than in the follicular phase. Ethnic differences also exist, with lower BGP levels occurring in African-Americans than in Caucasians. Similar to alkaline phosphatase, osteocalcin levels vary with age. Thus, children in active bone growth have higher circulating levels than adults, with a peak around the pubertal age for both sexes. Thereafter, serum osteocalcin stabilizes, until the fifth–sixth decade, when a significant rise occurs in females. This phenomenon is strictly linked to the menopausal ovarian failure, it is reproduced by oophorectomy, and is prevented by estrogen replacement therapy. Serum BGP returns toward premenopausal levels 15–20 years after the menopause.

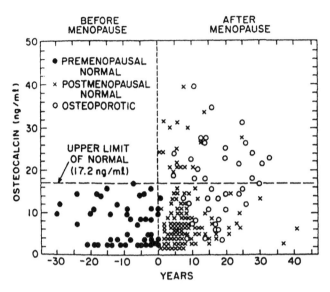

Fig. 5-1. Relationship between serum osteocalcin and age in normal and osteoporotic women. Premenopausal age was estimated by subtracting 50 to the chronological age of each patient. The osteocalcin upper limit of normal corresponds to the mean ± SD of premenopausal subjects. (Reproduced with permission from Yasumura AS, Aloia JF, Gundberg CM, Yeh J, Vasuani AN, Yuen K, LoMonte AF, Ellis KJ, Cohn SH: Serum osteocalcin and total body calcium in normal pre- and postmenopausal women and postmenopausal osteoporotic patients. J Clin Endocrinol Metab 64:681–685, 1987; © The Endocrine Society.)

However, the undercarboxylated fraction of osteocalcin increases constantly with age, reaching its highest levels (about 20% of total) in the seventh and eighth decades of life, probably indicating a reduced or abnormal osteoblast synthetic activity with aging. The menopause-related increase of serum osteocalcin is associated with a wider spread of values observed in subjects with osteoporosis, than in normal peers (Fig. 5-1). This reflects the wide spectrum of bone turnover characteristic of this disorder and accounts for the higher levels of osteocalcin observed in unselected osteoporotic women compared to healthy counterparts. Such a wide physiologic variability should be always borne in mind when interpreting serum BGP results, especially if the measurement is used to verify changes from previous conditions or to monitor the efficacy of treatment.

As noted above, BGP is increased in other metabolic bone diseases characterized by increased bone turnover, including Paget's disease of bone. However, probably because of the exceptionally high degree of cellular activity of this focal disorder, osteoblasts in areas affected by Paget's disease may reaccumulate some of the osteocalcin. Thus, the amount of osteocalcin entering the circulation may not be sufficient to cause a detectable increase (dilution effect). Consequently, this marker is not a good diagnostic index of pagetic activity, which can be more reliably estimated by alkaline phosphatase or markers of bone resorption.

Unlike other markers, osteocalcin levels decrease in conditions of low bone turnover, such as hypothyroidism, growth hormone deficiency, and inactive osteoporosis. Decreased osteocalcin levels are consistently found during corticosteroid treatment, and are correlated to the daily dose of the drug, thus representing a good index of the degree of steroid-induced suppression of bone formation. Therefore, osteocalcin can be either high, normal, or decreased, according to the rate of bone remodeling. Serum osteocalcin levels can be used to monitor the efficacy of antiresorptive medications, such as calcitonin or bisphosphonates in osteoporosis or other metabolic bone diseases. For example, a decline of serum BGP is observed after parathyroidectomy in primary hyperparathyroid patients. On the other hand, BGP increases after administration of 1,25-dihydroxycholecalciferol to osteoporotic subjects and patients with X-linked hypophosphatemic rickets, as well as in growth-deficient children treated with growth hormone.

Serum Type I Procollagen Propeptides

After the procollagen chains are synthesized by the osteoblast, part of the noncollagenous extension peptides are cleaved from both the carboxyl and amino termini, before collagen is assembled into fibrils. The resulting cleavage products, referred to as procollagen type I carboxyl- (PICP) and amino-terminal (PINP) propeptides, are then released into the extracellular fluid. Although a fraction of PINP may be incorporated into the bone matrix where it is released during bone resorption, the presence of both these collagen fragments in the circulation is directly related to deposition of new type I collagen, thereby representing a marker of bone formation. Although type I collagen is not exclusively produced in bone, the contribution of soft tissues to circulating PICP is quite small. These peptides are catabolized in the liver. Consequently they can be safely used in patients with renal failure, a slight advantage over BGP, although they should not be used in liver diseases.

PICP is a trimeric glycoprotein, with a molecular weight of about 100 kDa. Under reducing conditions, two similar but distinct subunits are produced, with a molar ratio of 2:1. PINP is an elongated triple-helical peptide smaller than PICP. Having only intrachain disulfide bonds, it is also more unstable than PICP, and it is probably the major substrate from which the many smaller circulating monomeric procollagen fragments are produced. Radio-immunoassays based on antibodies raised against either the N- or C-terminus of procollagen fragments have been developed but only PICP should be considered specific for bone formation.

Similar to osteocalcin, PICP is low in growth-deficient children and increases during treatment with growth hormone, suggesting a close correlation with bone growth. Menopause induces an ~20% increase in serum PICP concentration which is reversed by hormonal replacement therapy. Surprisingly, similar age-related changes have not been detected for PINP. Compared to PINP, PICP is more sensitive in detecting deviations from normal in patients with metabolic bone diseases, and correlates better with the calcium kinetics or bone histomorphometry. PICP is elevated in Paget's disease of bone where it correlates with serum bone-specific alkaline phosphatase and urinary hydroxyproline. Unfortunately, the degree of PICP changes that occur in pathologic conditions is not as large as for BGP or alkaline phosphatase. Although the reason for the relative insensitivity of the serum procollagen assays to physiologic oscillations in bone remodeling may rest on technical problems, these markers offer no clear advantage over alkaline phosphatase or BGP in routine clinical applications. Precise characterization of the circulating immunoreactive forms of type I procollagen may improve the sensitivity and specificity of these assays.

PARAMETERS OF BONE RESORPTION

During the process of bone resorption calcium salts are liberated from bone and, if not reutilized by the osteoblasts for new bone formation, they enter the circulation and are cleared by the kidney. Therefore, an increased bone turnover is usually associated with an increased urinary calcium output. Before the current biochemical markers were introduced, urinary calcium excretion represented the only humoral index available to estimate the rate of bone turnover. Although a moderate hypercalciuria should still be considered as a possible sign of increased bone remodeling rates, urinary calcium is under direct control of calciotropic hormones and it can only provide a rough estimate of bone remodeling.

Urine Hydroxyproline

One of the early steps in the posttranslational processing of procollagen chains consists in the hydroxylation of proline and lysine residues. This metabolic pathway is peculiar to collagen and essential for the protein to acquire its characteristic helix conformation. Hydroxyproline is therefore found almost exclusively in collagen, although a relatively minor amount of the amino acid is contained in other proteins, such as the C1q fraction of complement, which may account for up to 40% of total urine hydroxyproline in normal adults. This is one of the limiting factors to the specificity of this marker as index of bone turnover. Free hydroxyproline released into the circulation during collagen degradation cannot be reutilized for synthesis, and it is therefore filtered by the kidney. Although most of the amino acid is reabsorbed by the kidney and ultimately catabolized by the liver, the moiety of hydroxyproline present in the urine is strictly dependent on collagen turnover. Since collagen synthesis and breakdown occurs mostly—though not exclusively—in bone, measurement of urinary hydroxyproline can be used as a marker of bone turnover.

Total hydroxyproline in the urine is contributed to by three forms: the free amino acid, small peptides containing hydroxyproline, and larger hydroxyproline-containing polypeptides. The first two forms comprise the dialyzable fraction, which accounts for 90% of the total urinary hydroxyproline, and seems to originate from collagen degradation, thus representing the real bone resorption marker. The remainder 10%, nondialyzable hydroxyproline, is constituted by larger (5000–10,000 Da) polypeptides, and it is believed to derive from newly synthesized collagen fragments that are not incorporated into the matrix. As such, it reflects bone formation. Therefore, fractionation of hydroxyproline by dialysis theoretically can provide information on both formation and resorption processes. However, this time-consuming and poorly reproducible methodology has never gained widespread enthusiasm. For most clinical uses, measurement of total hydroxyproline has been employed as a parameter of bone resorption, an assumption that appears to be justified by the preponderant contribution of the dialyzable fraction to the total amino acid. Urinary hydroxyproline is well correlated with kinetic parameters of bone resorption, but not with the number of osteoclasts or resorption surfaces in histologic sections.

Hydroxyproline is measured in a urine sample using a colorimetric method after complete hydrolysis to free amino acid. Since urinary hydroxyproline is directly dependent on the glomerular filtration rate, the results are usually corrected by urinary creatinine excretion or clearance. Other correction factors have also been used, such as: body weight, body surface area, and bone mass of the radius. The latter would theoretically provide an index of bone resorption per volume unit of bone, but since bone density is usually measured at a single location, extrapolation of the index to the entire skeleton may be misleading. The excretion of hydroxyproline in a 24-h urine sample is heavily dependent on dietary collagen. Therefore the patient has to be instructed to follow a collagen-free diet for at least 2 days before urine collection, a burdensome procedure that has contributed to limit the applicability of the test. In alternative, hydroxyproline can be measured in a 2-h urine collection and corrected for creatinine after an overnight fast. The latter method seems to offer the same diagnostic value as the 24-h sample, with the advantage of being faster to perform and insensitive to dietary collagen.

Similar to other bone turnover markers, age- and sex-related changes in urinary hydroxyproline occur throughout life. Accordingly, this urine marker is higher in developing children than in adults, reaching a peak around the pubertal age, and decreasing thereafter. A postmenopausal increase of total hydroxyproline also occurs. Although the absolute amount of hydroxyproline in the urine decreases with age, probably reflecting a reduced bone mass,

renal function decreases too; consequently, the urinary hydroxyproline /
creatinine ratio slightly increases with age. Total urinary hydroxyproline is
elevated in metabolic bone diseases characterized by increased resorption,
such as Paget's disease of bone, metastatic bone tumors, hyperparathyroidism, as well as in hyperthyroidism and acromegaly. A decrease of hydroxyproline in these conditions indicates an improvement of the resorptive process, and it can be helpful to follow the response to treatment.

Urine Pyridinoline Cross-links of Type I Collagen

In order to stabilize the collagen fibrils in their characteristic trimeric structure, the polypeptidic chains have to be solidly bound together. Accordingly,
specific covalent cross-links are formed, both within the same triple-helical
chains and between different trimeric assemblies. These cross-links are initially aldehydic bonds between amino acid residues, mostly lysine, hydroxylysine, and histidine. In bone, cross-linking involves lysine and hydroxylysine, whereas in skin the major residue to be cross-linked is histidine. This
tissue-specific discrepancy offers the ground for the use of collagen cross-
links as markers of bone turnover. As the posttranslational cross-linking proceeds, it is believed that the reducible aldehydic bonds are converted to non-
reducible mature compounds. Two major cross-links are present in the matrix
of bone and cartilage, hydroxylysyl-pyridinoline and lysyl-pyridinoline, more
simply called pyridinoline (Pyr), and deoxypyridinoline (D-Pyr), respectively.
Thus, Pyr and D-Pyr cross-links bind adjacent collagen molecules via three
hydroxylysine residues (or two hydroxylysine and one lysine in the case
of D-Pyr), two of them originating from the short, terminal, nonhelical se-
quences and one from the helicoidal domain of the collagen molecule.

Whereas the concentration of Pyr and D-Pyr in connective tissues is very
low, D-Pyr is relatively abundant in bone and dentin, where it constitutes
about 22% of total hydroxypyridinoline cross-links. It is also present, although at much lower concentrations, in large vessels, tendons, and articu-
lar cartilage but it is absent from the skin. Because bone is by far the most
abundant source of collagen matrix and its turnover rate is markedly higher
compared to other connective tissues, Pyr and D-Pyr present in biological
fluids may be considered as deriving predominantly from bone. Both collagen cross-link metabolites are released from bone matrix during collagen
degradation into the circulation and are finally excreted into the urine. Pyr
and D-Pyr are not metabolized *in vivo,* and they cannot be reutilized. Therefore, they are excreted in the urine unchanged either free (~40%) or as peptide bound forms (~60%). Pyridinoline cross-links have several advantages
over urinary hydroxyproline, including their complete urinary excretion,
their absence in immature and skin collagen, and their insensitivity to dietary gelatin, suggesting that they are not absorbed by the intestine.

Pyridinoline cross-links can be measured in the urine by fluorometry after hydrolysis and purification by reverse-phase HPLC, utilizing the natural

fluorescence properties of the compounds. This assay is considered the gold standard for measuring cross-links, but it is inconveniently complex and time-consuming. Various immunoassays more suitable for routine use have been recently developed using antibodies which recognize either Pyr or D-Pyr free fractions, or epitopes in the cross-linked domains at both ends of the type I collagen molecule. The N-telopeptide-to-helix (NTX) end is the source of almost 60% of the D-Pyr in human bone collagen, as opposed to a 40% contributed by the C-telopeptide-to-helix (CTX) end. Collagen telopeptides are highly immunogenic and the considerable variability between the different collagen types provides the opportunity for developing collagen type-specific immunoassays.

Measurements are commonly performed in a 24-h urine sample. Initially, assessment of a fasting 2-h urine collection was also proposed, based on the observation that values obtained using the two collection methods usually agreed. However, a circadian rhythm in the excretion of D-Pyr has been observed in normal and osteoporotic female populations, with increased excretion rates at night. Thus, one must be very careful in interpreting a 2-h urinary value of the pyridinium cross-links, since daily variation of urinary pyridinoline cross-links are more pronounced than for any other marker. Similar to other markers, urinary Pyr and D-Pyr change with age. Accordingly, urinary Pyr and D-Pyr are higher in children than in adults; menopause causes a 2- to 3-fold raise of the urinary cross-links, and estrogen treatment restores the premenopausal levels. Interestingly, the Pyr/D-Pyr ratio (between 3 and 3.5 in normals) does not change with age, corroborating the hypothesis that in normal conditions most Pyr and D-Pyr result from bone resorption, and that metabolism of other connective tissues contributes little. Pyr and especially D-Pyr, correlate with bone turnover measured by calcium kinetics and bone histomorphometry.

Pyr and D-Pyr are elevated in a variety of conditions with increased bone turnover, such as: Paget's disease of bone, hyperparathyroidism, hyperthyroidism, but also in patients with osteoarthritis or rheumatoid arthritis, where the metabolites may also reflect cartilage breakdown. Interestingly, intravenous infusion of bisphosphonates to pagetic patients reduces urinary Pyr and D-Pyr within 24 h and before hydroxyproline decreases, suggesting that, unlike hydroxyproline, excretion of the cross-links is strictly proportional to bone resorption.

Free Pyr or D-Pyr concentration in the urine measured by the Pyrilink and Pyrilink-D assays, respectively, correlate well with total pyridinoline excretion measured by HPLC. Direct measurement of peptide-bound cross-links demonstrated that when bone turnover increases, the abundance of the peptide-bound moiety of cross-links is higher relative to free Pyr and D-Pyr, although both fractions increase in absolute terms. This is probably the result of a faster metabolic clearance of the free cross-links than peptide-bound cross-links, and perhaps a preferential release of the peptide-bound forms during bone resorption. The monoclonal antibody used in the Osteomark NTX assay recognizes epitopes in the NTX cross-linking domain of human type I collagen. The participation of α_2 (I) collagen chains to the cross-linking at the N-terminus of the molecule should confer a higher bone specificity to NTX compared to CTX assays. Urine NTX concentration measured by this quite specific assay is markedly increased after menopause and in patients with hyperthyroidism or Paget's disease of bone. The antibody used in the Crosslaps assay is raised against a synthetic octapeptide corresponding to a fragment of the C-telopeptide sequence of α_1 (I) collagen chain, in which one lysine residue is involved in the cross-linking. This should ensure minimal cross-reactivity with other types of collagen. Urine CTX levels are increased after menopause in almost one-third of all postmenopausal women, and in patients with Paget's disease of bone, hyperparathyroidism, and hyperthyroidism. They correlate well with urine hydroxyproline and free D-Pyr.

An immunoassay that measures type I collagen C-telopeptides (ICTP) in the serum has been recently tested. Because the helical part of the α-chains is strongly conserved among different types of collagen, the specificity of this assay in reflecting bone resorption may not be the best, and degradation products of collagen type II and/or III may cross-react with the antibody used in this assay. In fact, human studies have not corroborated the clinical usefulness of this parameter. Although serum ICTP levels correlate with histomorphometric measurements of bone turnover in iliac crest biopsies and increase in patients with bone metastases, they are not high in Paget's disease of bone, nor does hormonal replacement therapy significantly alter serum ICTP. On the contrary, anabolic steroids that presumably decrease bone resorption and increase collagen synthesis increase serum ICTP concentration. Overall, serum ICTP can be considered a good index of collagen turnover, but a less sensitive marker of bone resorption.

Other Bone Resorption Markers

Urine Hydroxylysine Glycosides. As described above, lysine residues are hydroxylated, along with proline, during the posttranslational processing of collagen α chains. Therefore, the excretion of hydroxylysine residues should also reflect bone matrix breakdown. Theoretically, measuring this amino acid in the urine should provide a more selective index of bone resorption, as compared to hydroxyproline, in view of the fact that hydroxylysine glycosides are entirely excreted into the urine. Moreover, glycosylation of lysine residues during collagen processing is at a certain extent tissue-specific. Accordingly, β-1-galactosyl-hydroxylysine (GHL) is a prevalent product of bone collagen, whereas α-1,2-glycosyl-galactosyl-hydroxylysine (GGHL) is more specific of skin collagen. Thus, the GHL/GGHL ratio should provide an index reflecting the metabolic activity of either tissue. Indeed, the ratio is increased in Paget's disease of bone, and decreased in burn patients with extensive skin damage. Age-related oscillations of urinary GHL, similar to those observed for hydroxyproline, have also been described. Correlations between GHL, or GHL/GGHL ratio and rate of bone loss have also been reported in osteoporotic females, but the data have remained confined to preliminary reports on small sample populations. An additional problem is represented by the fact that the pattern of glycosylated hydroxylysine excretion in normal subjects and in patients with Paget's disease of bone is not entirely consistent with an exclusive bone origin, suggesting an alternative source of these modified amino acid (i.e., C1q), or "abnormal" glycosylation profiles in this particular disorder. The method for measuring hydroxylysine glycosides is also complex, based on HPLC separation of the different forms, which contributes to the limitations of this marker for routine clinical applications.

Plasma Tartrate-Resistant Acid Phosphatase. The enzymatic properties of acid phosphatase are similar to those of alkaline phosphatase, except that its pH optimum is acidic. Acid phosphatase activity, like alkaline phosphatase, is present in various tissues, including bone, prostate, spleen, erythrocytes, and platelets. The bone isoenzyme is only expressed by osteoclasts and it is used to characterize their phenotype. Therefore, acid phosphatase represents a potentially specific marker of osteoclastic activity and bone resorption. Osteoclast acid phosphatase can be separated from the other isoenzymes because it is the only form resistant to tartrate. Indeed, tartrate sensitivity is the characteristic exploited for the identification of prostate acid phosphatase, the other major isoform present in the circulation in normal individuals. Tartrate-resistant acid phosphatase activity (TRAP) has been found to be elevated in primary hyperparathyroidism, in patients with bone metastases, and other disorders associated with high bone turnover, such as Paget's disease of bone, osteomalacia, hyperthyroidism, and glucocorticoid treatment. Consistent with other bone resorption markers, TRAP increases after menopause and after oophorectomy. Although a negative correlation has been reported between TRAP and bone mineral density in osteoporotic patients, the instability of TRAP activity in frozen plasma samples and the presence of enzyme inhibitors in serum are potential drawbacks which have limited the diffusion of this marker in clinical applications. New immunoassays using monoclonal antibodies that specifically recognize the bone isoenzyme of TRAP should help define the diagnostic value of this marker for osteoclast activity.

MARKERS OF BONE TURNOVER IN OSTEOPOROSIS

Biochemical Markers as Diagnostic Tools

The rapid development of new and more sensitive biochemical markers of bone turnover has spawned numerous studies in the attempt to define the potential clinical usefulness of these markers in the management of patients with osteoporosis. Indeed, the ability to predict bone loss and more importantly the risk of new fractures by a simple biochemical test would simplify the diagnostic process in these patients with significant cost savings. However, the usefulness of these biochemical indices for diagnostic and therapeutic decisions in osteoporosis is still limited. The major limitations to a more widespread applicability of biochemical markers of bone turnover stem from the inadequacy of a single biochemical test to reliably predict bone loss and fracture risk in individual patients, the relatively high day-to-day variability, and the cost and availability of the test itself. Whereas these theoretical considerations may be quite difficult to overcome, it seems likely that a lower cost—perhaps by inclusion of one of these parameters in auto-mated analyzers—would immediately expand the use of bone remodeling markers to other important clinical questions including, but not limiting to, monitoring patient compliance and short-term response to therapy.

In the previous sections, we have discussed how bone turnover slowly but gradually increases in both sexes with age, and that in women a post-menopausal transient is overimposed on the age-related increase. There is a wide individual variability in the magnitude of the postmenopausal increase of bone turnover, depending on the individual genetic background and lifestyle habits, and this variability translates into a similar histologic hetero-geneity. Several studies in recent years have reported negative correlations between markers of bone turnover and bone density, a correlation that be-comes stronger with aging. One of these studies demonstrated that the con-tribution of bone turnover—assessed by a battery of biochemical markers—accounts for only 10% of bone density in perimenopausal women, but its importance increased with age, explaining up to 50% of bone density vari-ance after age 75 (Fig. 5-2). The relatively low contribution of bone turnover to bone loss until later in life underscores the limited predictive value of a single determination of bone turnover for bone loss in the majority of post-menopausal women. This notion becomes rather obvious if one considers that a biochemical marker reflects the cellular activity at that particular mo-ment in time, whereas bone mass is the result of a lifelong process of mod-eling and remodeling. Better correlations have been observed between a single measurement of a biochemical marker and rates of bone loss in the following years in postmenopausal populations (Fig. 5-3). Unfortunately, the correlation coefficients are invariably very low, and the high standard errors of estimate preclude extrapolation to individual patients.

Combination of different markers, such as fasting Pyr or D-Pyr, urinary hydroxyproline, and serum BGP, increases the predictive value for subse-quent bone loss in postmenopausal women. Multiple markers and one bone mineral density measurement have been used to construct an algorithm as a screening procedure to diagnose osteoporosis and estimate future bone loss. Based on this method, postmenopausal women could be classified as "fast losers" if the predicted bone loss was >3% per annum, or "slow losers" if the predicted loss was below that limit. In a 12-year follow-up of a rela-tively large group of postmenopausal women, Hansen and co-workers (1991) observed that despite identical bone mass at baseline, "fast losers"

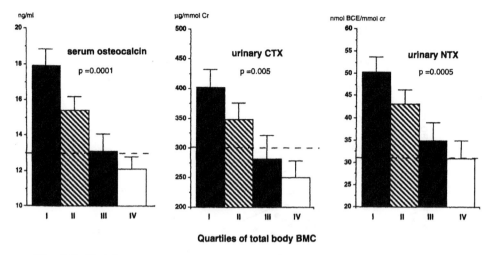

Fig. 5-2. High bone turnover is associated with low bone density in elderly post-menopausal women. A cohort of women postmenopausal for 20 years or more were stratified in quartiles based on bone mineral density. Quartiles 1 and 4 are statistically different ($p < 0.05$). (Reproduced from Garnero P, Sornay-Rendu E, Chapuy MC, Delmas P: J Bone Miner Res 1996; 11:337–349; with permission of the American Society for Bone and Mineral Research.)

lost 50% more bone than those identified as "slow losers." Although such results need to be confirmed in larger populations, combining one baseline bone mass measurement with a battery of bone turnover markers is a plausible approach to estimate the rate of bone loss and thus identify those menopausal women who are at highest risk of developing osteoporosis.

Another albeit less critical limitation to the clinical application of biochemical markers is the day-to-day variability. Although indices of bone formation and resorption may fluctuate randomly in osteoporotic patients, subjects with high-turnover forms of osteoporosis generally continue in this category. Furthermore, repeated measurements of bone formation and resorption markers for several months in osteoporotic women yield relatively low individual long-term coefficients of variation. Thus, with the refinement of the technical aspects of these biochemical assays, it is reasonable to expect that this source of variability may be controlled in the near future.

The possibility of using biochemical markers of bone turnover to predict the risk of hip fracture represents the ultimate standard for assessing the validity of these parameters as diagnostic tools in osteoporosis. Only with the development of more sensitive assays, in particular pyridinoline cross-links, have such studies been undertaken. In a recently published European longitudinal survey on a large number of postmenopausal women, higher baseline values of urinary CTX and free D-Pyr were observed in subjects

ROBERTO CIVITELLI

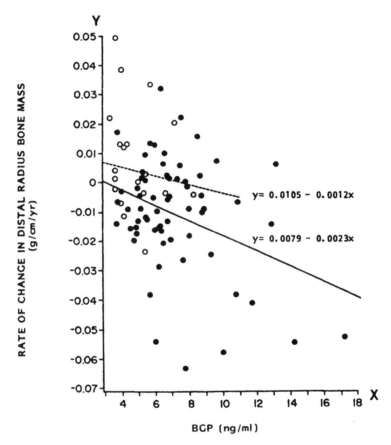

Fig. 5-3. Individual rates of distal radius bone mass changes as a function of serum osteocalcin (BGP) in 84 early perimenopausal (open circles and dashed line) and postmenopausal (closed circles and line) women. The weighted regression for the entire
group is $y = 0.0122 - 0.0027x$. (Reproduced from Slemenda CW, Hui SL, Longcope C,
Johnston CC Jr: The Journal of Clinical Investigation 80:1261-1269, 1987, by copyright permission of the American Society of Clinical Investigation.)

who sustained a hip fracture in the following 2 years, as compared to age-
matched women who did not experience hip fractures (Fig. 5-4). Quite
surprisingly, only those two bone resorption markers were significantly elevated in this cohort, as NTX and bone formation markers (BGP, bone-
specific alkaline phosphatase) were not different between cases and controls.
Furthermore, only women with CTX or D-Pyr above the premenopausal
range had a 2-fold relative risk of hip fractures, independently of bone density and physical performance. As one would expect, those women with

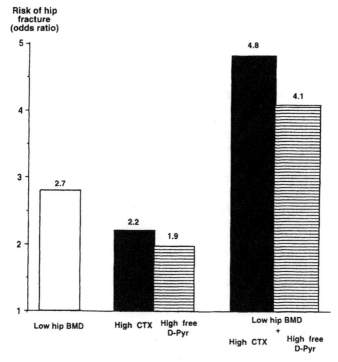

Fig. 5-4 Markers of bone resorption can predict risk of hip fracture in elderly women. A cohort of 126 women (mean age 82.5 years) who sustained a hip fracture during a 22-month observation period were matched with 2 controls who did not fracture. Serum levels of CTX and free D-Pyr were collected at the beginning of the period of observation. Calculated odds ratios (95% confidence interval) are 2.2 (1.3–3.6) and 1.9 (1.1–3.2) for CTX and D-Pyr, respectively. (Reproduced from Garnero P, Hausherr E, Chapuy MC, Marelli C, Grandjean H, Muller C, Cormier C, Breart G, Meunier PJ, Delmas PD: J Bone Miner Res 1996; 11:1531–1538, with the permission of the American Society for Bone and Mineral Research.)

bone density in the osteoporotic range (more than 2.5 standard deviations below the average of young individuals) and high CTX or D-Pyr had the worse prognosis, with more than 4-fold increased fracture risk. Another interesting finding emerged from the same European study. Elderly institutionalized women who sustained a hip fracture during a 18-month follow-up period, had significantly higher circulating levels of undercarboxylated BGP at baseline than control subjects without fractures. In these elderly women, having a low hip bone density and high undercarboxylated BGP increased the risk of hip fracture 5-fold, although the variability was high. This interesting observation may reflect a vitamin K deficiency, which is not uncommon in elderly patients with hip fracture. These results are rather appealing, but it remains to be seen how the additional information provided by biochemical markers can affect clinical decisions that could otherwise be made on the basis of bone density only.

Application to Treatment Selection and Monitoring

Patients with accelerated bone turnover tend to loose bone at a faster rate than those with normal turnover, therefore they should be the best candidates for antiresorptive therapy. The first demonstration of this hypothesis came from a study from our group. Postmenopausal women with high turnover osteoporosis responded to subcutaneous salmon calcitonin therapy with significant gains in vertebral bone density, as opposed to no changes observed in individuals with normal bone remodeling. Similar results have been later reported by other investigators who were able to predict the response to calcitonin therapy in terms of changes in bone density by baseline measurements of biochemical markers of bone turnover. At least two studies have shown that response to estrogen is also dependent on levels of bone turnover markers at the initiation of treatment. Although the potential relevance of these studies is rather obvious, the clinical impact of effective screening methods to identify subjects that would better respond to antiresorptive therapy relies entirely on our ability to precisely predict bone loss by a single assessment of bone turnover, an issue that is far from being settled. Moreover, because antiresorptive therapies depress bone remodeling, prediction of response to these type of medications is by definition limited to short-term changes. The current lack of valid alternatives to antiresorptive medications for the treatment of osteoporosis further reduces the importance of bone turnover markers for clinical decisions on osteoporosis therapy. However, this conclusion may change in the near future with the introduction of anabolic agents that can uncouple the remodeling cycle by stimulating bone formation.

Hormone replacement therapy decreases both resorption and formation markers to premenopausal levels within 3 to 6 months of therapy. Even more rapid responses have been obtained with bisphosphonates. Treatment with alendronate dose-dependently decreases serum BGP and urinary Pyr after only 6 weeks of treatment. Thus, biochemical markers can rapidly report changes in bone turnover in response to antiresorptive therapy. After withdrawal of hormonal replacement therapy, bone turnover markers return to pretreatment values within 3 months, the same time that is necessary to detect a decrease following initiation of therapy. Considering the relatively low compliance to hormone replacement therapy, the potential clinical utility of these parameters for monitoring adherence to therapy is immediately obvious. If the current costs could be lowered, it is very likely that physicians may find biochemical markers of bone turnover very useful in this regard.

On the other hand, whether bone turnover markers can be used to predict response to treatment is still very controversial. Studies on antiresorptive therapies in osteoporotic populations have shown that in average subjects who gain bone mass also experience larger declines in bone turnover indices compared to individuals that exhibit less exuberant responses in terms of bone density. However, the differences between groups are usually very small and within the precision error of the biochemical tests performed. Although it is true that the correlation between changes in bone turnover markers and changes in bone density is much stronger when the two variables are assessed at the same time, such finding has no real relevance for a diagnostic use of these biochemical tests as predictors of a therapeutic response. One study has recently reported a weak correlation between changes in one bone resorption marker, NTX, and changes in bone density after 12 months of estrogen replacement, with a 2.2-fold higher likelihood of gaining bone density in 1 year of treatment in those subjects who experienced a 30% decline of NTX, relative to those who exhibited lesser or no changes (Fig. 5-5). However, 57% of the treated patients with less than 30% decrease in NTX still improved or maintained bone density, and the predictive value of NTX was significant for changes in vertebral but not proximal femur bone density. Although these data are of extreme importance and

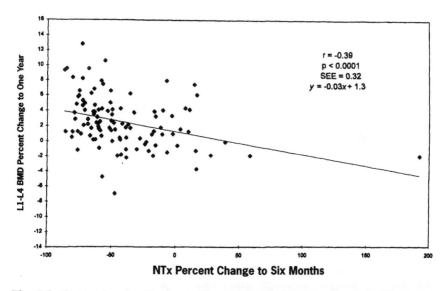

Fig. 5-5 Changes in urine N-telopeptide cross-links of type I collagen (NTX) are correlated to changes in bone density in women treated with estrogen replacement. Urine NTX was measured at baseline and after 6 months of therapy. Spine bone density was followed at 6-month intervals for up to 2 years while women were receiving either estrogen or placebo. (Reprinted from Am J Med, 102, from Chesnut CH III, Bell NH, Clark GS, Drinkwater BL, English SC, Johnston CC Jr, Notelovitz M, Rosen CJ, Cain DF, Flessland KA, Mallinak NJS: Hormone replacement therapy in postmenopausal women: Urinary N-telopeptide of type I collagen monitors therapeutic effect and predicts response of bone mineral density, 29–37. Copyright 1997, with permission from Excerpta Medica Inc.)

significance, they should not be construed to suggest that two serial measurements of a bone turnover marker at baseline and 3–6 months into treatment would yield the same information about the efficacy of antiresorptive therapy as it can be obtained by measuring bone density in 1 or 2 years. This is certainly unwarranted for such therapies as estrogen replacement or bisphophonates which induce net increases in bone density. Bone turnover markers may theoretically be more suitable for monitoring patients on other forms of treatment for osteoporosis, in particular calcitonin or raloxifene. Recent data indicate that these two medications substantially reduce fracture risk in spite of relatively small changes of bone density, and that reduction of bone remodeling may account in part for their beneficial effect. Accordingly, assessment of bone turnover could be advocated as a reasonable method for monitoring compliance and efficacy of these two therapeutic regimens in reducing bone remodeling rates.

In summary, fundamental limitations still preclude the generalized application of biochemical markers of bone turnover to monitor treatment response. Even the most recent and promising studies confirm poor correlations with changes in bone density, high standard errors of estimates, and most importantly, high variability of the marker relative to the changes induced by treatment. In the vast majority of postmenopausal women, values of bone turnover markers fall within the normal range, and in fact, only a minority of subjects (<30%) experience high bone turnover and "fast" bone loss. Because the precision error of the currently used biochemical markers of resorption, especially those measured in the urine, exceeds the magnitude of the change that occurs during treatment, in most cases it is impossible to distinguish between treatment effect and day-to-day individual variability. Averaging more than one measurement may reduce this variability, but the problem remains that individual responses cannot be inferred by group behaviors, and in the clinical setting it is the individual patient that counts.

FUTURE DIRECTIONS

The improved sensitivity and precision of biochemical markers of bone turnover have expanded their potential applications in the management of osteoporotic patients, although many issues regarding their use and interpretation remain controversial. While BGP and bone-specific alkaline phosphatase currently represent the most specific markers of bone formation, there are still plenty of indications for continuing to use the less sensitive, but simple and inexpensive total alkaline phosphatase, especially in very high bone turnover conditions. The increasing knowledge on the structure and regulation of other noncollagenous bone matrix proteins, such as bone sialoprotein and proteoglycans, all synthetic products of osteoblasts, will direct the future development of bone formation markers. The clinical usefulness in therapeutic decisions involving bone resorption inhibitors has pushed most of the recent efforts toward bone resorption markers. The development of assays for measurement of pyridinoline cross-links represents the most important step in this direction and has provided a valuable marker whose clinical use will certainly increase in the near future.

Although markers of bone turnover most likely will never supplant bone densitometry as the standard diagnostic tool for the diagnosis and management of osteoporosis, accumulating data seem to suggest that these biochemical tests may in the future become part of the diagnostic approach to the osteoporotic patient. Defining the most appropriate therapeutic intervention and monitoring treatment effectiveness are two critically important niches for the use of biochemical markers of bone turnover in this condition. It is foreseeable that with the increasing available therapeutic options and the mounting prevalence of osteoporosis in elderly populations these two niches will rapidly expand.

SUGGESTED READING

Beardsworth LJ, Eyre DR, Dickson IR: Changes with age in urinary excretion of lysyl- and hydroxylysyl pyridinoline, two new markers of bone collagen turnover. J Bone Miner Res 5:671–676, 1990.

Calvo MS, Eyre DR, Gundberg CM: Molecular basis and clinical application of biological markers of bone turnover. Endocr Rev 17:333–368, 1996.

Chesnut CH III, Bell NH, Clark GS, Drinkwater BL, English SC, Johnston CC Jr, Notelovitz M, Rosen CJ, Cain DF, Flessland KA, Mallinak NJS: Hormone replacement therapy in postmenopausal women: Urinary N-telopeptide of type I collagen monitors therapeutic effect and predicts response of bone mineral density. Am J Med 102:29–37, 1997.

Christiansen C, Hassager C, Riis BJ: Biochemical markers of bone turnover. In Avioli LV, Krane SM (eds.): Metabolic Bone Disease and Clinically Related Disorders, San Diego, Academic Press, 1998, pp. 313–326.

Civitelli R, Gonnelli S, Zacchei F, Bigazzi S, Vattimo A, Avioli LV, Gennari C: Bone turnover in postmenopausal osteoporosis: Effect of calcitonin treatment. J Clin Invest 82:1268–1274, 1988.

De La Piedra C, Torres R, Rapado A, Curiel MD, Castro N: Serum tartrate-resistant acid phosphatase and bone mineral content in postmenopausal osteoporosis. Calcif Tissue Int. 45:58–60, 1989.

Delmas PD, Steiner D, Wahner HW, Mann KG, Riggs BL: Serum bone gla-protein increases with aging in normal women: Implications for the mechanism of age-related bone loss. J Clin Invest 71:1316–1321, 1983.

Delmas PD, Demiaux B, Malaval L, Chapuy MC, Meunier PJ: Serum bone Gla-protein is not a sensitive marker of bone turnover in Paget's disease of bone. Calcif Tissue Int 38:60–61, 1986.

Delmas PD, Gineyts E, Bertholin A, Garnero P, Marchand F: Immunoassay of pyridinoline crosslink excretion in normal adults and in Paget's disease. J Bone Miner Res 8:643–648, 1993.

Eastell R, Simmons PS, Colwell A, Assiri AMA, Burritt MF, Russel RGG, Riggs BL:

Nyctohemeral changes in bone turnover assessed by serum bone Gla-protein concentration and urinary deoxypyridinoline excretion: Effects of growth and ageing. Clin Sci 83:375–382, 1992.

Ebeling PR, Atley LM, Guthrie JR, Burger HG, Dennerstein L, Hopper, JL, Wark, JD: Bone turnover markers and bone density across the menopausal transition. J Clin Endocrinol Metab 81:3366–3371, 1996.

Garnero P, Delmas PD: Assessment of the serum levels of bone alkaline phosphatase with a new immunoradiometric assay in patients with metabolic bone disease. J Clin Endocrinol Metab 77:1046–1053, 1993.

Garnero P, Delmas PD: Biochemical markers of bone turnover. Applications for osteoporosis. Endocrinol Metab Clin North Am 27:303–323, 1998.

Garnero P, Hausherr E, Chapuy MC, Marcelli C, Grandjean H, Muller C, Cormier C, Breart G, Meunier PJ, Delmas PD: Markers of bone resorption predict hip fracture in elderly women: The EPIDOS prospective study. J Bone Miner Res 11:1531–1538, 1996.

Garnero P, Sornay-Rendu E, Chapuy MC, Delmas PD: Increased bone turnover in late postmenopausal women is a major determinant of osteoporosis. J Bone Miner Res 11:337–349, 1996.

Hansen, MA, Kirsten O, Riis BJ, Christiansen C: Role of peak bone mass and bone loss in postmenopausal osteoporosis: A 12 years study. Br Med J 303:961–964, 1991.

Hanson DA, Weis MA, Bollen AM, Maslan SL, Singer FR, Eyre DR: A specific immunoassay for monitoring human bone resorption: Quantitation of type I collagen cross-linked N-telopeptides in urine. J Bone Miner Res 7:1251–1258, 1992.

Hassager C, Jensen LT, Johansen JS, Riis BJ, Melkko J, Paedenphant J, Risteli L, Christiansen C, Risteli J: The carboxy-terminal propeptide of type I procollagen in serum as a marker of bone formation: The effect of nandrolone decanoate and female sex hormones. Metabolism 40:205–208, 1991.

Hoogkinson A, Thompson T: Measurement of the fasting urinary hydroxyproline: creatinine ratio in normal adults and its variations with age and sex. J Clin Pathol 35:807–811, 1982.

Moro L, Mucelli RS, Gazzarrini C, Modricky C, Marotti F, De Bernard B: Urinary β-1-galactosyl-O-hydroxylysine (GH) as a marker of collagen turnover of bone. Calcif Tissue Int 42:87–90, 1987.

Riis BJ, Overgaard K, Christiansen C: Biochemical markers of bone turnover to monitor the bone response to postmenopausal hormone replacement therapy. *Osteoporosis Int* 5:276–280, 1995.

Rosen CJ, Chesnut CH III, Mallinak NJS: The predictive value of biochemical markers of bone turnover for bone mineral density in early postmenopausal women treated with hormone replacement or calcium supplementation. J Clin Endocrinol Metab 82:1904–1910, 1997.

Schlemmer A, Hassager C, Jensen SB, Christiansen C: Marked diurnal variation in urinary excretion of pyridinium cross-links in premenopausal women. J Clin Endocrinol Metab 74:476–480, 1992.

Slemenda CW, Hui SL, Longcope C, Johnston CC Jr: Sex steroids and bone mass. A study of changes about the time of menopause. J Clin Invest 80:1261–1269, 1987.

Slovik DM, Gundberg CM, Neer RM, Lian JB: Clinical evaluation of bone turnover by serum osteocalcin measurements in a hospital setting. J Clin Endocrinol Metab 59:228–230, 1984.

Stepán JJ, Pospícal J, Presl J, Pacovsky V: Bone loss and biochemical indices of bone remodeling in surgically induced postmenopausal women. Bone 8:279–284, 1987.

Stepán JJ, Silinkova-Malkova E, Havranek T, Formankova J, Zichova M, Lachmanova J, Strakova M, Broulik P, Pacovsky V: Relationship of plasma tartrate resistant acid phosphatase to the bone isoenzyme of serum alkaline phosphatase in hyperparathyroidism. Clin Chim Acta 133:189–200, 1983.

Uebelhart D, Schlemmer A, Johansen JS, Gineyts E, Christiansen C, Delmas PD: Effect of menopause and hormone replacement therapy on the urinary excretion of pyridinium cross-links. J Clin Endocrinol Metab 72:367–373, 1991.

Vergnaud P, Garnero P, Meunier PJ, Breart G, Kamihagi K, Delmas PD: Undercarboxylated osteocalcin measured with a specific immunoassay predicts hip fracture in elderly women: The EPIDOS Study. J Clin Endocrinol Metab 82:719–724, 1997.

Yasumura AS, Aloia JF, Gundberg CM, Yeh J, Vaswani AN, Yuen K, Lo Monte AF, Ellis KJ, Cohn SH: Serum osteocalcin and total body calcium in normal pre- and postmenopausal women and postmenopausal osteoporotic patients. J Clin Endocrinol Metab 64:681–685, 1987.

6 Calcium, Vitamin D, and Bone Metabolism

Bess Dawson-Hughes

INTRODUCTION

The effect of increasing calcium and vitamin D intakes on patterns of bone loss and fracture rates has been studied extensively over the past 8 to 10 years. Most of these studies have been carried out in postmenopausal women, a group at high risk for osteoporosis. This chapter will review current evidence concerning the extent to which intakes of these nutrients influence bone metabolism, describe a rapid approach to estimating intake, and suggest approaches to help individual patients meet the recent intake recommendations.

CALCIUM AND VITAMIN D METABOLISM

Calcium and vitamin D intakes alter calcium regulating hormone levels and bone mass. As shown in Fig. 6-1, an inadequate intake of either of these nutrients results in a reduced amount of absorbed calcium and subtle lowering of the circulating ionized calcium concentration. The latter then stimulates the release and raises the blood level of parathyroid hormone (PTH). The PTH returns the blood calcium level to normal by decreasing the renal excretion of calcium, by promoting the activation of vitamin D (which stimulates calcium absorption), and by promoting bone resorption. In most older people, bone remodeling is uncoupled in favor of bone resorption. Because of this, the PTH-induced increase in bone remodeling in such individuals

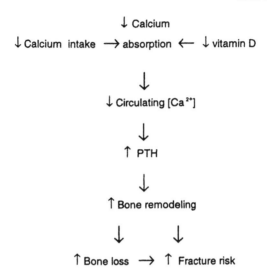

Fig. 6-1. Effect of calcium deficiency on PTH and bone turnover. (From Ross EM: Nutrition in Clinical Care 1(2), 1998.)

results in an increased rate of bone loss. Over time, this is associated with an increase in fracture risk. There is also evidence now that an increase in the bone turnover rate, independent of its effect on bone mineral density (BMD), increases risk of fracture.

With aging the efficiency of calcium absorption declines. The relative calcium deficiency leads to an age-related increase in circulating PTH levels and to the other changes described in Fig. 6-1. Calcium supplementation in older men and women will produce a sustained reduction in circulating levels of PTH and in biochemical markers of bone turnover. In one study, high dose supplementation (1600 mg per day) in older women lowered serum PTH and biochemical markers of bone resorption to levels observed in young healthy women.

Several changes in vitamin D physiology occur with aging. Vitamin D is formed in the epidermal layer of the skin on exposure to ultraviolet rays of the sun. With aging, the skin thins and contains less of the vitamin D substrate, 7-dehydrocholesterol. As a result, the efficiency of vitamin D production in skin declines severalfold. There is some evidence that vitamin D absorption also declines with aging, although this point is somewhat controversial at this time. It is widely recognized that circulating levels of 25-hydroxyvitamin D, the best index of clinical vitamin D status, decline with aging.

Vitamin D levels fluctuate with the season in much of the temperate zone. In the summer, optimal 25-hydroxyvitamin D levels can be maintained with exposure of the face and arms to sunlight for as little as 10 to 15 min per day. In the winter, however, the ultraviolet β rays needed to promote vita-min D synthesis do not reach Earth's surface. As a result, individuals are de-pendent on dietary sources for their vitamin D during the winter. People who are institutionalized or who wear sunscreen on a regular basis will of course be dependent on dietary sources for vitamin D year-round. In Bos-ton, at latitude 42° N, 25-hydroxyvitamin D levels decline in older men and women by about 25% from summer to winter. The wintertime decline can be prevented with vitamin D supplements of 400 to 800 international units (IU) per day.

BONE LOSS AND FRACTURES

A number of investigators have tackled the subject of how much calcium and vitamin D is needed to minimize bone loss. Most studies have been con-ducted in women because they are at greatest risk for osteoporotic fractures. In the early menopause, as estrogen levels decline, rates of bone loss accel-erate. The average rate of loss for healthy early postmenopausal women is about 3% of the skeletal mass per year. After 5 to 8 years, the rate of loss de-clines to an average of about 1% per year. It is recently appreciated that bone loss continues and may even accelerate in very elderly men and women.

The effect of calcium and vitamin D on rates of bone loss in early post-menopausal women has been widely studied. It is very clear at this time that calcium and vitamin D supplementation will not prevent estrogen deficiency related bone loss. However, the rate of loss at skeletal sites rich in cortical bone can be modestly attenuated with calcium supplementation. At trabecu-lar rich skeletal sites such as the spine however, supplementation may im-prove BMD initially by lowering the bone turnover rate, but after the first year of treatment, no further benefit to BMD is seen. A recent meta-analysis indicated that in early postmenopausal women, BMD gains from hormone replacement therapy (HRT) were significantly greater in women who also took calcium supplements than they were in women who took HRT without added calcium. In this analysis, the calcium-supplemented women had an average intake of about 1200 mg per day compared with half that intake level in the unsupplemented women. This analysis underscores the impor-tance of an adequate calcium intake in women taking HRT.

Many randomized controlled trials examining the effect of added calcium and or vitamin D on rates of bone loss have been conducted in women who were 6 or more years beyond menopause. In these women, calcium fairly consistently lowers rates of bone loss at cortical and trabecular rich skeletal sites. Several studies have tested supplementation with vitamin D. In one such study all women were placed on calcium supplements and the women were then randomized to either a vitamin D supplement or a placebo. The vitamin D supplemented women had lower rates of bone loss than did the women taking calcium only. More recently, combined calcium and vitamin D supplementation has been shown to reduce bone loss in healthy women age 65 and older.

A number of recent studies have looked at the effect of calcium and/or vitamin D on incidence of low trauma fractures. Of four relatively small calcium intervention studies, three identified fewer fractures in the calcium group than in the placebo group. A fourth study found no difference in fracture rates in the two arms. Two large vitamin D intervention studies have been conducted in very elderly men and women in northern Europe. In one, an annual intramuscular injection of vitamin D reduced fracture rates. In the other, an oral supplement of 400 IU of vitamin D per day had no effect on fracture rates. There are several reports of the effects of combined calcium and vitamin D supplementation on fracture rates. In very elderly French women residing in nursing homes, combined supplementation with 1200 mg of calcium and 800 IU of vitamin D daily significantly lowered hip and other nonvertebral fracture rates. These women had usual dietary calcium intakes of about 500 mg per day and very low 25-hydroxyvitamin D levels. The effect of combined supplementation was evaluated recently in active men and women, age 65 and older, who resided at home in Boston. Subjects who took 500 mg calcium and 700 IU vitamin D daily had less bone loss and fewer clinical fractures over the 3-year study period than those who took placebo.

RECOMMENDED INTAKES OF CALCIUM AND VITAMIN D

In 1997, the Institute of Medicine of the National Academy of Sciences revisited the subject of recommended intakes of calcium and vitamin D for Americans. A scientific panel was appointed and assigned the task of interpreting the available literature in order to provide evidence-based intake recommendations. The calcium intakes recommended for adults were based on the amount that promoted the maximal calcium retention, defined as the most positive calcium balance that could be achieved as a result of increasing calcium intake. Other criteria included the intake needed to minimize bone loss and to reduce fracture incidence. The vitamin D intake recommendations were based on the amount needed to prevent a wintertime decline in the serum 25-hydroxyvitamin D level and to minimize rates of bone loss. The recommended calcium and vitamin D intakes, designated as adequate intakes, are shown in Table 6-1. It is notable that a calcium intake of 1200 mg per day is recommended for postmenopausal women independent of their use of HRT. The calcium intakes are increased above those recommended in 1989. These represent the first increases since the initial recommendation of the Academy of 800 mg per day in 1941. Vitamin D intake recommendations have changed over the years but comparative values for 1989 were lower, as shown in Table 6-1.

For the first time, the National Academy identified safe upper limits for

**TABLE 6-1. National Academy of Sciences Intake
Recommendations—Past and Present**

Age	Calcium, mg/day		Vitamin D, IU/day	
	1989	1997	1989	1997
31-50	800	1000	200	200
51-70	800	1200	200	400
71+	800	1200	200	600
Safe upper limit[a]		2500		2000

[a]Pertains to healthy men and women in all of these age groups.

calcium and vitamin D. This important addition acknowledges the potential for consuming an excess of these nutrients, given the increasing popularity of fortified foods and nutraceuticals. To identify the safe upper limit, three potential adverse events were considered: kidney stones, hypercalcemia with renal insufficiency (milk alkali syndrome), and the interference of calcium with the absorption of other essential nutrients. High intakes of dietary calcium have actually been associated with a lower incidence of first kidney stone formation. In contrast, high intakes of calcium from supplements may increase the risk of kidney stones by up to 20% in women, although no dose effect has been identified. Of the three potential adverse effects, data adequate for identification of a dose response relationship were available only for the milk alkali syndrome. Based on this syndrome, the critical intake was defined as 5 g of calcium per day. Application of a safety factor of 2 then resulted in a safe upper limit of 2500 mg per day.

For vitamin D, the safe upper limit was defined as the highest intake known not to cause hypercalcemia. This upper limit, after application of a safety factor, was set at 2000 IU per day. For each of these nutrients, there is a large margin between the recommended intake and safe upper limit.

The new recommended intakes far exceed actual median intakes in the US population of adult men and women. Based on the 1994 U.S. Department of Agriculture Continuing Survey of Food Intakes of Individuals, the median calcium intake of men was 857 mg per day at ages 31 through 50, 708 mg at ages 51 through 70, and 702 mg at ages 71 and above. These values are 30 to 40% below the recommended intake of 1200 mg per day. Women in the United States consume less than half of the needed calcium. In the same survey, the median intake of women was 606 mg per day for ages 31 through 50, 571 mg for ages 51 through 70, and 501 mg for women ages 71 and above.

Comparable national intake data for vitamin D are not available but several estimates by individual investigators place the mean intake at around 150 to 200 IU per day. As with calcium, vitamin D intake is far below levels recommended for men and women aged 51 and older.

**TABLE 6-2. Calcium Content
of Selected Dairy Foods**

Dairy Food	Serving Size, oz	Ca Content, mg
Skim milk	8 (or 1 cup)	302
Yogurt		
Plain	8	415
With fruit	8	345
Cheese	1	150[a]
Cottage cheese	4	63
Ice cream	4	88

[a]Varies from 100 to 200, with harder cheeses containing more calcium.

ASSESSING INDIVIDUAL CALCIUM AND VITAMIN D INTAKES

In order to make appropriate recommendations to individual patients, it is first necessary to assess their current intake of calcium and vitamin D. Because nearly 75% of dietary calcium in the United States is of dairy food origin, total intake can be approximated by assessing an individual's average intake from dairy foods (see Table 6-2) and then adding about 250 mg to cover calcium from all other dietary sources. A similar process can be easily undertaken for vitamin D. In one large study of healthy postmenopausal women, the percentages of total dietary vitamin D derived from specific foods was 67% from milk, 13% from margarine, and 20% from other sources including cereals.

MEETING INTAKE REQUIREMENTS

Several approaches can be taken to increase calcium and vitamin D intakes to recommended levels. It is preferable to meet the calcium and vitamin D intake requirements by adjusting the diet. For those who can not or will not consume the needed amounts of these nutrients from natural and fortified foods, supplements may be needed. When using supplements, several issues must be considered including the choice of a specific calcium salt, the dosage and schedule, and the safety of the supplement.

A number of comparative studies of the absorbability of calcium supplements have been performed with somewhat inconsistent results. Under similar experimental conditions, calcium absorption from the different supplements ranges from about 25 to 35%. Calcium carbonate is most widely

**TABLE 6-3. Supplement Contents and
Absorbability of Calcium from 500 mg
Calcium Load without a Meal[a]**

Supplement	Calcium Content, mg/g of Supplement	Fractional Absorption, %
Carbonate	400	35
Acetate	230	32
Citrate	210	35
Lactate	130	34
Gluconate	90	27

[a] Absorption measured by a variety of methods.

consumed because it has the highest proportion of calcium per gram weight of supplement (Table 6-3).

The purity of calcium supplements, at least with respect to lead content has been examined. The lead content, normalized to 800 mg of calcium, is low in refined supplements (less than 1 mcg), but ranges from 4 to 11 mcg for dolomite, products labeled natural source, and bone meal. For comparison, there is less than 1 mcg of lead in an equivalent amount of milk. Although the risk of lead intoxication from many of these supplements is low (because co-ingestion with calcium limits the absorbability of the lead), refined calcium supplements are nonetheless preferred because of their very low lead content.

With regard to supplement dosage, for the most efficient absorption, single doses should not exceed 500 to 600 mg. Thus for those needing more than this amount, the dosage should be split.

The timing of supplement use is important for calcium carbonate. Absorption is greater and more consistent when this supplement is taken with or after meals. Some scientists generally recommend a supplement dose at bedtime on the grounds that it will suppress the nocturnal rise in PTH and/or reduce nocturnal bone resorption. Direct evidence for a better result from supplements taken at night rather than at other times of the day is not currently available.

CONCLUSION

Based on a substantial body of evidence, the National Academy of Sciences recently raised recommended intakes of calcium and vitamin D for adults. Usual intakes in the United States are currently far below recommended intakes. For individual patients, it is important to estimate their current intake and develop a tailored approach to help them meet their calcium and vitamin D intake requirements. Broad implementation of these recommendations should significantly reduce osteoporotic fracture rates in the United States.

SUGGESTED READING

Aloia JF, Vaswani A, Yeh JK, Ross PL, Flaster E, Dilmanian FA: Calcium supplementation with and without hormone replacement therapy to prevent postmenopausal bone loss. Ann Intern Med 120:97–103, 1994.

Bruce DG, St John A, Nicklason F, Boldswain PRT: Secondary hyperparathyroidism in patients from western Australia with hip fracture: Relationship to type of hip fracture, renal function, and vitamin D deficiency. JAGS 47:354–359, 1999.

Burgoin BP, Evans DR, Cornett JR, Lingard SM, Quattrone AJ: Lead content in 70 brands of dietary calcium supplements. Am J Public Health 83:1155–1160, 1993.

Chapuy MC, Arlot ME, Doboeuf F, Brun J, Crouzet B, Arnaud S, Delmas PD, Meunier PJ: Vitamin D_3 and calcium to prevent hip fractures in elderly women. N Engl J Med 327:1637–1642, 1992.

Chapuy MC, Schott AM, Garnero P, Hans D, Delmas PD, Meunier PJ, and EPIDOS Study Group: Healthy elderly French women living at home have secondary hyperparathyroidism and high bone turnover in winter. J Clin Endocrinol Metab 81:1129–1133, 1996.

Curhan GC, Willett WC, Speizer FE, Spiegelman D, Stampfer MJ: Comparison of dietary calcium with supplemental calcium and other nutrients as factors affecting the risk for kidney stones in women. Ann Intern Med 126:497–504, 1997.

Dawson-Hughes B: Calcium, vitamin D, and risk of osteoporosis in adults: Essential information for the clinician. Nutr Clin Care 1:63–70, 1998.

Dawson-Hughes B, Harris SS, Krall EA, Dallal GE: Effect of calcium and vitamin D supplementation on bone density in men and women 65 years of age or older. N Engl J Med 337:670–676, 1997.

Elders PJM, Netelenbos JC, Lips P, van Ginkel FC, Khoe E, Leeuwenkamp OR, Hackeng WHL, van der Stelt PF: Calcium supplementation reduces vertebral bone loss in perimenopausal women: A controlled trial in 248 women between 46 and 55 years of age. J Clin Endocrinol Metab 73:533–540, 1991.

Heaney RP, Smith KT, Recker RR, Hinders S: Meal effects on calcium absorption. Am J Clin Nutr 49:372–376, 1989.

Heshmati HM, Khosla S, Burritt MF, O'Fallon WM, Riggs BL: A defect in renal calcium conservation may contribute to the pathogenesis of postmenopausal osteoporosis. J Clin Endocrinol Metab 83:1916–1920, 1998.

Jacques PF, Felson DT, Tucker KL, Mahnken B, Wilson PWF, Rosenberg IH, Rush D: Plasma 25-hydroxyvitamin D and its determinants in an elderly population sample. Am J Clin Nutr 66:929–936, 1997.

McKane WR, Kholsa S, Egan KS, Robins SP, Burritt MF, Riggs BL: Role of calcium intake in modulating age-related increase in parathyroid function and bone resorption. J Clin Endocrinol Metab 81:1699–1703, 1996.

New SA, Bolton-Smith C, Grubb DA, Reid DM: Nutritional influences on bone mineral density: A cross-sectional study in premenopausal women. Am J Clin Nutr 65:1831–1839, 1997.

Nieves JW, Komar L, Cosman F, Lindsay R: Calcium potentiates the effects of estrogen and calcitonin on bone mass: Review and analysis. Am J Clin Nutr 67:18–24, 1998.

Prince RL, Dick IM, Lemmon J, Randell D: The pathogenesis of age-related osteoporotic fracture: Effects of dietary calcium deprivation. J Clin Endocrinol Metab 82:260–264, 1997.

Reid IR, Ames RW, Evans MC, Gamble GD, Sharpe SJ: Long-term effects of calcium supplementation on bone loss and fractures in postmenopausal women: A randomized controlled trial. Am J Med 98:331–335, 1995.

Standing Committee on the Scientific Evaluation of Dietary Reference Intakes: Dietary reference intakes: calcium, phosphorus, magnesium, vitamin D, and fluoride. Institute of Medicine. Washington, D.C.: National Academy Press, 1997.

Sheikh MS, Santa Ana CA, Nicar MJ, Schiller LR, Fordtran JS: Gastrointestinal absorption of calcium from milk and calcium salts. N Engl J Med 317:532–536, 1987.

Thomas MK, Lloyd-Jones DM, Thadhani RI, Shaw AC, Deraska DJ, Kitch BT, Vamvakas EC, Dick IM, Prince RL, Finkelstein JS: Hypovitaminosis D in medical inpatients. N Eng J Med 338:777–783, 1998.

7 Estrogens and Selective Estrogen Receptor Modulators for Prevention and Treatment of Osteoporosis

Robert Lindsay

Louis V. Avioli

INTRODUCTION

One of the significant events that occurs ubiquitously among women as they age is the relatively sudden cessation of ovarian function. The outward appearance of this is the cessation of menses or the menopause. A similar precipitous cessation of testicular function does not occur in males, although there is a slow and gradual decline in testicular function with age. The loss of ovarian function is accompanied by significant changes in skeletal homeostasis with consequent loss of bone tissue. The effects are marked and occur in every female and the consequences are more significant than those of any of the other lifestyle and nutritional factors generally considered to be important in the pathogenesis of osteoporosis. The resulting bone loss is more obvious in cancellous (also known as trabecular) bone, but occurs in all parts of the skeleton, increasing the risk not only of vertebral fracture, but also fractures of hip, distal radius, and other bones. Although only 20% of the skeleton is composed of cancellous bone, excessive loss of this skeletal component accounts for the dramatic differences in vertebral fractures between the sexes which are from 5–10 times more common among women, whereas hip fractures are only twice as common in females as they are in males.

In premenopausal women, bone mass is essentially stable, although bone loss may be minimal at some skeletal sites prior to the onset of menopause. The postmenopausal acceleration of bone loss is probably self-limiting in most individuals, although the factors controlling its rate and duration are neither well defined nor understood. Since not all women develop fractures, it seems likely that either peak bone mass (or rather bone mass at the onset of ovarian failure) or rate and duration of subsequent loss are determinants of the likelihood of fractures. A single determination of bone mineral density predicts the risk of future fracture in postmenopausal women and probably does so at all ages, although the majority of the data have been obtained in older populations. The accumulated data suggest that initial bone mass is important. However, results of recent studies which indicate that increased bone remodeling is independently associated with the risk of fracture suggest that rates of loss are also important. In cancellous bone, the greater the extent of rapid bone turnover, the more likely it is that trabecular architecture will be disturbed as bone mass is lost (Fig. 7-1). It is the combination of loss of bone mass and the associated disturbance in architecture that cre-

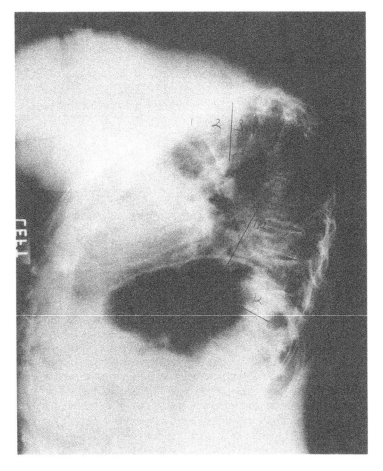

Fig. 7-1. Dorsal kyphosis in a patient with severe vertebral osteoporosis.

ates the steep gradient between risk of fracture and declining bone mass which, when producing vertebral fractures, results in an increased mortality rate particularly from chronic pulmonary disease.

ESTROGEN DEFICIENCY

Menopause is associated with a loss of virtually all endocrine functions of the ovary with the exception of some continuing secretion of androgen by the ovarian stroma. The role of androgens of ovarian origin in determining the rate of bone loss in postmenopausal women is still not clear, but may in part account for the increased severity of the bone loss which has been observed in women who have suffered surgical ovariectomy when compared to those with a simple clinical menopause.

In most women, a gradual decline in ovarian function begins between 35 and 45 years of age with increasing anovulatory cycles and menstrual irregularity. Ovarian function generally ceases by age 55 in a great majority of individuals (mean in the United States is 51 years). In some studies, there is a relationship between the age of menopause and the risk of fracture, although this is not an unusual finding. Such relationships are more difficult to find with the fractures that occur in later life such as hip fracture. It is not clear if this occurs because hip fractures are equally dependent on falls which occur with increasing frequency among the elderly, particularly among women, or simply is indicative of the lesser ability of elderly women to accurately date the onset of the menopause.

The alterations of circulating estrogenic and androgenic steroids after the menopause are shown in Table 7-1. Although there are declines in all steroids, the decline is significantly less and not statistically significant for testosterone (Table 7-1). The predominant estrogen secreted by the ovary of premenopausal women is 17β-estradiol. In postmenopausal women, there is a greater decline in estradiol than in estrone, which then becomes the

TABLE 7-1. Changes in Circulatory Steroids after the Menopause

	Premenopausal	Postmenopausal
Estradiol	0.05 ± 0.005	0.013 ± 0.001
Estrone	0.08 ± 0.01	0.06 ± 0.01
Testosterone	0.41 ± 0.02	0.25 ± 0.03 (ns)[a]
Dihydrotestosterone	0.29 ± 0.02	0.15 ± 0.02
Androstenedione	1.90 ± 0.01	0.50 ± 0.04

Reprinted with permission from the American College of Obstetricians and Gynecologists (Abraham GE, Maroulis GB: Effect of endogenous estrogens on serum prendenolone, cortisol, and androgens in postmenopausal women. Obstet Gynecol 45:271–274).

[a]ns, not significant

dominant estrogen, although estrone also circulates in reduced amounts when compared to the premenopausal state. Thus, total estrogen levels decline and the ratio of estradiol/estrone decreases. In many tissues, estrone can be converted to estradiol intracellularly which binds to either the alpha (α) or the recently discovered beta (β) estrogen receptor. Progesterone, secreted mainly by the corpus luteum after ovulation, declines as the number of anovulatory cycles increase as menopause approaches. In the postmenopausal woman, the adrenal gland becomes the principal source of sex steroids including small quantities of progesterone. Conversion of androgens (androstenedione and testosterone) of adrenal origin to estrogen (estrone and estradiol) occurs primarily in fat and muscle; the bulk of these tissues available for aromatization probably determines the circulating concentration of estrogen in postmenopausal women. The rate of bone loss in periand postmenopausal women has been shown to be correlated with circulating estrogen levels and in some studies appears also to be related to circulating androgen levels.

These alterations in the availability of the "sex" steroids and their metabolism are accompanied by marked changes in skeletal homeostasis. Increased activation of bone remodeling and, perhaps, an increased activity or the number of osteoclasts results in net loss of bone tissue as the deficit between bone resorption and formation in each remodeling cycle increases. Consequently, there is a slight increase in serum and a more significant increase in urinary calcium. Intestinal calcium absorption also declines as bone becomes a more significant contributor to the available extracellular calcium pool. This increase in skeletal turnover is evidenced by increased circulating levels of bone specific alkaline phosphatase and bone derived osteocalcin, biomarkers which are related to the formation of new bone. Urinary excretion of hydroxyproline, deoxypyridinoline, and the telopeptides of either the amino or carboxyl terminus of the collagen molecule also rises the latter reflecting the increased resorption of bone which characterizes increased skeletal turnover. Increased serum phosphorus and more efficient resorption of phosphate in the renal tubule suggest reduced parathyroid activity at least in the early postmenopausal period. Changes in parathyroid hormone across the menopause have not been universally documented, although dramatic increments can occur later in the calcium–vitamin D deficient, more elderly postmenopausal female.

If the primary skeletal defect that results from ovarian failure is increased bone remodeling, then the following sequence of events would be expected (Fig. 7-2). Estrogen loss results in an increase in the efflux of calcium from the skeleton to blood and causes a reduction in the secretion of parathyroid hormone. This is followed by a reduction in the hydroxylation of 25-hydroxyvitamin D_3 to its active metabolite, 1,25-dihydroxyvitamin D_3, a process that occurs in the kidney and which is controlled principally by parathyroid hormone and serum calcium. The consequence would be reduced efficiency of vitamin D dependent calcium absorption. There would also be an increase in the excretion of calcium in urine and an increase in the tubular reabsorp-

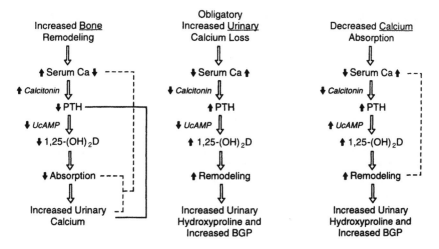

Fig. 7-2. Postulated impairments in hormonal control of calcium metabolism that might occur after menopause and account for the observed changes in mineral and skeletal homeostasis.

tion of phosphate. Although reduced circulating parathyroid hormone and 1,25-dihydroxyvitamin D_3 would lower the drive to increase bone remodeling, this is compensated by an increased skeletal sensitivity to parathyroid hormone in the postmenopausal woman as a result of estrogen loss. Alternative hypotheses used to explain bone loss includes an obligatory increase of urinary calcium loss and/or a defect in calcium absorption, which would tend to raise both blood parathyroid hormone and 1,25-dihydroxyvitamin D_3 (Fig. 7-2). In fact, the major change that occurs across the menopause appears to be increased skeletal remodeling, although there may be concommitant changes in renal or intestinal calcium handling as a consequence of loss of estrogen.

Whereas receptors for estrogen have been found in cells of the osteoblast lineage derived from bone, they have not been consistently identified in osteoclasts. This supports the hypothesis of a direct action of sex steroids on skeletal bone formation although we recognize that it is still questionable as to whether studies on bone cells *in vitro* mimic those events which occur in the intact skeleton responding to estrogen. Estrogen receptors are present in other cells in the bone marrow and in bone marrow fibroblasts. Thus, estrogen effects on the skeleton are also likely to be mediated by one of the many cytokines secreted by mononuclear cells, fibroblasts, or marrow cellular constituents. Implicated molecules include growth factors such as transforming growth factor beta (TGF β), insulin-like growth factors, a variety of interleukins, and prostaglandins.

Although the precise mechanism of estrogen action on the skeleton is still conjectural at best, estrogen deficiency clearly increases the activation of bone remodeling and the progressive loss of skeletal tissue. The bone remodeling cycle, a preventive maintenance process that maintains the skeleton at a relatively youthful chronological age (and may also be responsible for the repair of bone microdamage) is a process that occurs in discrete places on the skeleton surface. The process is characterized by a recruitment of bone resorbing cells to the bone surface, which, after they remove a predetermined amount of skeletal tissue, leave and are replaced by mononuclear cells whose purposes may well be to prepare the surface for new bone formation. The mononuclear cells in turn are replaced by teams of osteoblasts which replace the bone that has been removed with new organic material called "osteoid." The latter is subsequently mineralized as an extracellular process. In the best of all possible worlds, during the normal skeletal remodeling process the amount of bone that is laid down equals the amount of bone that is removed. In the postmenopausal woman, as a consequence of estrogen deficiency, there is an increase in the number of remodeling sites present which produces a transient increase in bone loss. There may also be an imbalance between resorption and formation in favor of the former which contributes to a more long-term deficit of bone mass. As a consequence of these distubances in bone remodeling there is loss of bone tissue, disturbance of skeletal architecture, and an increase in the risk of fracture.

THE EFFECT OF ESTROGEN

The administration of estrogens to postmenopausal women produces effects in mineral homeostasis which are the exact converse of those skeletal events which characterize ovarian failure. Estrogen replacement causes a reduction in bone remodeling with a consequent reduction in the circulating levels or the excretion of bone remodeling biomarkers (i.e., blood osteocalcin, bone specific alkaline phosphatase; and urinary deoxypyridinoline, N-telopeptides, C-telopeptides). These effects are accompanied by a conservation of bone mass (Fig. 7-4). In most circumstances, when bone loss is progressing in an unrelentless fashion and estrogens are introduced, there is a transient increase in bone density in the order of 5–6% in the spine and 2–3% in the femoral neck. This increase in bone mineral density which occurs over the first 1 to 2 years of estrogen treatment is presumed to be related to the reduction in the activation of new remodeling cycles. Bone mineral density becomes stable after 1–2 years of estrogen treatment and, in most individuals, remains stable for at least several years provided adequate doses of estrogen are supplied (Fig. 7-3). Although most clinical trials have relatively short duration (2–3 years), information gained from long-term observations suggests that estrogen treatment ultimately stabilizes bone mass. However, some observational data from epidemiological studies suggest that after very long-term estrogen use, there may be a gradual loss of bone that is more obvious in the femoral neck than at other skeletal sites. This effect may be related to the other pathophysiological events that alter bone re-

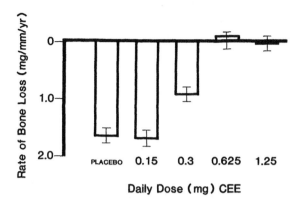

Fig. 7-3. The effects of various doses of conjugated equine estrogen on bone loss. Allocation to treatment program was done randomly using placebo and 0.15-, 0.30-, 0.625-, and 1.25-mg doses of conjugated estrogens. Rate of loss was calculated for each individual over a 2-year period. Reprinted with permission from the American College of Obstetricians and Gynecologists (Lindsay *et al.*: Obstet Gynecol 63:759–763, 1984).

modeling in the aging individual, including gradually declining calcium absorption, impaired vitamin D intake or sunlight exposure, reduced physical activity, and progressive increments in bone resorbing cytokines. Consequently, the increased risk of hip fracture in women appears to be created by the compounding effects of age and its biological sequelae and the menopause with its loss of hormones. In addition, since there is an increased risk of falling among the elderly, that may be more obvious in women than in men (at least up to the ninth decade), it is not surprising that preservation of bone mass produced by past estrogen use does not eliminate the risk of hip fractures, most of which occur following a fall.

Estradiol, estrone, and esterified and conjugated estrogens given by the oral route all produce reductions in bone remodeling and preservation of bone mass. Estriol by virtue of its pharmacokinetic and pharmacodynamic behavior must be given in excessively large doses to produce a "therapeutic" skeletal effect. Estradiol given by the transdermal percutaneous or subcutaneous route is similarly effective provided sufficient estrogen is administered and patient compliance established. When estradiol is given by the transdermal route, assessments of circulating estradiol suggest that circulating levels between 50 and 100 pg/ml are sufficient to produce an adequate skeletal response. As illustrated in Fig. 7-3, the minimum effective dose of conjugated equine estrogens required to prevent bone loss completely is 0.625 mg/day. Recent studies in women age >65 years do reveal that continuous therapy with conjugated equine estrogens, 0.3 mg/day, and medroxyprogesterone, 2.5 mg/day, combined with adequate calcium and vitamin D resulted in a preservation of bone mass. To date, these observations have not been made in younger postmenopausal populations with any degree of consistency. Attempts to reduce the side effects of estrogens while still maintaining efficacy has resulted in a short-term (6 months) open-label randomized study of postmenopausal women with transdermal patches designed to deliver 25 mg of β-estradiol daily (which were worn for 7 days before replacement). When compared to an untreated control group, bone mineral density in the lumbar spine and femoral neck of the estradiol treated group increased whereas that of the control group decreased. Once again, short-term studies of this nature require extension in order to guarantee that these effects of low-dose estrogens are not transient before this approach can be recommended as potentially effective in reducing bone loss and preventing fracture. A recent evaluation of the control clinical trials that have been performed using estrogens suggest that the apparent increased sensitivity to esterified estrogens is a phenomenon related to the introduction of calcium supplementation routinely into clinical trials. Evaluation of the control clinical trials with estrogen or other bone "stabilizing" drugs reveals that in studies performed without calcium supplements estrogens have less effects on bone mass than in those studies in which estrogen had been given together with calcium supplementation (Fig. 7-4). Thus the addition of calcium per se may explain the differences between the clinical trial results, rather than intrinsic differences in the different estrogens used in these studies. Since there is a greater incidence of endometrial hyperplasia and cancer associated with unopposed estrogen therapy, it is mandatory that progestins are also administered to women with intact uteri.

Estrogen therapy appears to prevent bone loss at all skeletal sites (Table 7-2) including the important sites of fracture, that is, the spine and the femoral neck. One of us (R.L.) has observed that, after 10 years of estro-

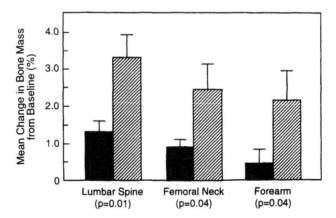

Fig. 7-4. Mean ($\pm$ SEM) annual percentage change in bone mass at the lumbar spine, femoral neck, and forearm in postmenopausal women treated with estrogen alone ($\square$, total average calcium intake 563 mg/day) compared with women treated with estrogen and calcium ($\blacksquare$, total average calcium intake 1183 mg/day). (Courtesy of R. Lindsay.)

TABLE 7-2. Frequency of Edentia by Use of ERT and by Age[a]

Age Group, years	Frequency of Edentia, %				
	No ERT	ERT	Duration of ERT, years		
			≤3	4–14	15+
<70	3.8	7.8	9.1	7.7	6.1
70–74	11.0	6.3	7.2	6.2	6.1
75–79	12.5	6.9	7.5	6.7	6.9
80–84	14.1	8.4	11.8	7.9	5.7
85–89	14.2	10.5	15.7	6.7	8.1
90+	16.9	13.0	15.3	13.6	8.8
Age-adjusted RR	1.00	0.64	0.85	0.57	0.49
95% CI	—	0.51–0.79	0.64–1.13	0.43–0.76	0.36–0.68

[a]ERT indicates estrogen replacement therapy; RR, relative risk; CI, confidence interval. Source: Arch Intern Med 155:2325, 1995. Copyright 1995, American Medical Association.

gen therapy, bone mass was 24% higher in the lumbar vertebrae than that observed in placebo treated individuals and 12% greater in the femoral neck. Prospective data confirmed that this preservation of bone mass also resulted in a decrease in the incidence of vertebral fracture. Data from a variety of epidemiological studies demonstrated that estrogen exposure reduced the risk of vertebral and hip fracture and fractures of the distal radius by approximately 58% (Table 7-3). Moreover, recent data from *the Study of Osteoporotic Fractures* suggest that the earlier that estrogen treatment is initiated, the greater the effect on fracture incidence, and that the effects on

TABLE 7-3. Studies Indicating a Reduction in Fractures with Estrogen Use

Author	Journal	Year	Fracture[a]	Relative Risk
Hutchinson	Lancet	1979	H, C	
Johnson	Am J Public Health	1981	H	
Krieger	Am J Epidem	1982	H	0.5
Paganini-Hill	Ann Intern Med	1981	H	
Weiss	N Engl J Med	1980	H, C	0.4
Williams	Obstet Gynecol	1982	H, C	
Kiel	N Engl J Med	1987	H	0.35
Ettinger	Ann Intern Med	1985	All	
Lindsay	Lancet	1980	V	ns[b]
Naessen	Ann Intern Med	1990	H	0.79

[a]H, hip; C, Colles'; V, vertebral.
[b]ns, not stated.

fracture incidence are more obvious in those individuals who continue to take estrogen long-term. The accumulated data confirm the conclusions drawn from the studies in which changes in bone mineral density had been used as an effective response. In those studies where there was primarily preservation of bone mass, the earlier estrogen intervention was initiated in the postmenopausal period, and the greater was the ultimate beneficial effect. In addition, several studies have now shown that the effects of estrogen are lost after the hormone therapy is discontinued. In this context, discontinuing estrogen is akin to a medical ovariectomy; as would be expected in either circumstance, bone turnover increases again and bone mass is lost. The longer that process continues, the more likely it is that bone density in that population will become similar to an untreated postmenopausal population. Consequently, we can assume that the effect of estrogens on fractures will be gradually lost.

Estrogen intervention can also be used in the treatment of elderly patients with established osteoporosis who are actively losing bone mass. In these patients, estrogen intervention produces the same transient increase in bone mass observed in the early postmenopausal years. However, of the few controlled clinical trials that have been performed in elderly populations beneficial effects have been noted in bone mineral density (BMD) (Fig. 7-5). The results of one relatively short-term controlled clinical trial with transdermal estrogens in a small elderly population also suggested a reduction in the risk of vertebral fracture of approximately 60%. Although the majority of epidemiological data support the conclusion that one would expect to find a reduction in the risk of fractures in the more aged osteoporotic population as a result of estrogen treatment, it would be comforting to have a large-scale controlled clinical trial confirming the fracture efficacy and determining its magnitude. Finally, there is accumulating data demonstrating that the risk

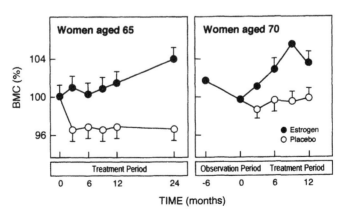

Fig. 7-5. Bone loss is prevented in postmenopausal women independent of age. (Courtesy of R. Lindsay.)

of alveolar bone loss and edentulous is significantly lower in women on replacement hormone therapy than in those who were untreated.

In general, the addition of a progestin that is used to protect the endometrium in the postmenopausal population on estrogen therapy neither adds nor negates the effects of estrogen on the skeleton. Results from the Progestin Estrogen Prevention Intervention Study (PEPI) indicate that neither micronized progesterone nor medroxyprogesterone acetate given cyclically or continuously modify estrogens effects on the skeleton. Results of one study, however, suggests that norethindrone acetate, a 19-nortestosterone derivative, may produce an additive effect when combined with estrogen. Although the addition of testosterone in small doses to estrogen may also produce an additive effect on the skeleton, the data require confirmation in large-scale studies wherein fracture outcome is evaluated to determine whether or not such combinations produced a greater effect on fracture incidence than estrogens alone.

MECHANISM OF EFFECT

As noted above, the precise mechanism(s) whereby estrogen withdrawal increases the rate of bone turnover is still ill-defined since the direct and indirect effects of estrogen on the skeleton are still to be established. There is certainly a decline in bone turnover and perhaps also a reinstatement of the balance between formation and resorption during estrogen therapy. Estrogens modify the activity of osteoblast-like cells *in vitro*, although immunohistochemical studies demonstrate a heterogeneity of estrogen receptor expression in osteoblast populations. Estrogens also produce modifications in cell growth or the synthesis and secretion of growth factors such as TGF β. The current dictum is also consistent with the hypothesis that cytokines must be responsible (at least in part!) for the bone loss resulting from estrogen deficiency. A few observations also support the hypothesis that the "bone sparing" effect of estrogen is due to the ability of the hormone to increase osteoclastic instability and apoptosis.

OTHER (NONSKELETAL) EFFECTS OF ESTROGEN

Estrogens are potent hormones that affect many systems of the body and as such it is not surprising that estrogen prescription is associated with effects other than those on the skeleton. Although the most common reason for estrogen prescription in the postmenopausal population is menopausal symptoms, estrogens also produce effects on the cardiovascular and urogenital systems, breast, and uterus. Whereas the unwanted uterine effects can be minimized with concomitant progestin treatment, there is currently no effective approach to minimize the estrogen-induced changes in breast tissue other than lowering estrogen doses and decreasing the total exposure to estrogens.

There is universal agreement that cardiovascular disease is the number one cause of mortality in the postmenopausal population. Although epidemiological data suggest that estrogen use reduces the risk of cardiovascular disease by about 50%, a variety of controlled studies have recently been designed to evaluate long-term effects of estrogens on cardiovascular disease in female populations. The Heart and Estrogen/Progestin Replacement Study (HERS) was designed as a randomized, double-blind placebo-controlled trial to test the effect of daily use of conjugated equine estrogens plus medioxyprogesterone acetate on the combined rate of nonfatal myocardial infarction and congestive heart disease among postmenopausal women with established heart disease. The results, obtained from a population with an average follow-up of 4.1 years, demonstrated no significant differences between the placebo or hormone-treated groups in either the incidence of myocardial infarction or cardiovascular morbid events. Since there were fewer morbid cardiovascular events in the hormone-treated groups in the latter years of the study, it was considered appropriate for women already receiving hormone treatment to continue taking the drug.

The potential mechanism(s) of the cardio-protective effect of estrogens is not entirely clear. Estrogens reduce low density lipoproteins and especially when given orally increase HDL, specifically the HDL-2 subfraction. These alterations are generally accepted as beneficial, but probably account only in part for the magnitude of estrogen effects recorded from epidemiological studies since direct effects of estrogens on myocardial activity and coronary artery dynamics have been demonstrated. In any event, we will probably receive much more definitive data detailing the relationship between estrogen replacement and coronary heart disease from the Women's Health Initiate Study (WHI) which is currently being explored in 25,000 women in the United States during a 9-year observation period. Although there is a tendency to ascribe a therapeutic effect of estrogens on cognitive function and dystrophic brain diseases such as Alzheimer's dementia, these identifications are poorly conjectural at this time.

SELECTIVE ESTROGEN RECEPTOR MODULATOR DRUGS

Currently fewer than 25% of the nearly 50 million postmenopausal women are on hormone replacement therapy. The complexity of estrogen prescription, bleeding episodes, coupled with the fear of breast cancer, often make the decision regarding hormone replacement therapy a difficult one for both physician and patient (Table 7-4). By 1 year, less than 50% of patients continue treatment. In a recent U.S. survey of 495 postmenopausal women 50–74 years of age it was noted that sociodemographic facts such as region and education were more often associated with the use of hormone replacement

**TABLE 7-4. Main Reasons Given
for Discontinuing Hormone
Replacement Therapy**

Reason	Number of Subjects
Bleeding episodes (withdrawal or irregular)	79 (44.8%)
Fear of cancer	51 (28.9%)
Dislike of drug use everyday	10 (5.6%)
Others	36 (20.4%)
Total	176 (100%)

Karakoc B *et al.*: Menopause 5:102–106, 1998.

therapy than clinical factors. Thus, long-term use of estrogen, likely required to obtain the maximum effect on disease outcomes is often not achieved. The realization that certain agents could produce antiestrogen effects in some tissues, while producing estrogen agonist responses in others has led to the concept of "designer estrogens"or "tissue selective estrogens," for which the term selective estrogen receptor modulators (SERM) has been established. SERM drugs which are currently marketed or in clinical development include the triphenylethylenes (tamoxifen and its derivatives toremifene, droloxifene, and idoxifene) and the benzothiophene, raloxifene (Fig. 7-6).

Recent developments in molecular biology have begun to shed light on the mechanisms by which SERM drugs may produce tissue dependent estrogen agonist or antagonist effects. These agents appear to produce cellular responses through interaction with the estrogen receptors. The more recent demonstration of a second estrogen β receptor, which shares common structural and functional characteristics with the α receptor although its gene resides on a different chromosome from the classic α receptor, initially led to the hypothesis that tissue distributions of the receptor isoforms could explain the tissue selective actions of estrogen-like substances. This hypothesis was subsequently regarded as simplistic since many tissues express both receptors. A second hypothesis, that is, that binding of each agent to the receptor creates a different molecular configuration of the ligand receptor complex with resulting differences in the capacity to bind to estrogen response elements or even binding to DNA components which are not classically estrogen receptors, is more intriguing since this paradigm for tissue selectivity implies that each ligand might produce a different spectrum of effects.

Clomiphene and tamoxifen were two of the original SERM drugs which were used for many years for different clinical purposes, that is, the induction of ovulation and prevention of secondary breast cancer respectively. Both drugs prevent bone loss in ovariectomized animals, and in addition tamoxifen reduces bone loss in postmenopausal women (Fig. 7-7). Raloxifene, a benzathiophene SERM, was originally developed for breast cancer

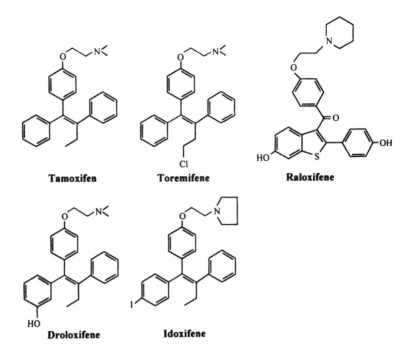

Tamoxifen   Toremifene   Raloxifene

Droloxifene   Idoxifene

Fig. 7-6. Various SERM compounds that are phenylethylene derivatives and structurally related to tamoxifen. Raloxifene is a benzothiopene derivative and is a SERM with clinical effects similar to those of tamoxifen, except in the uterus, where it is a pure antiestrogen. (Adapted from Goldstein: Selective estrogen receptor modulators: A new category of therapeutic agents for extending the health of postmenopausal women. Am J Obstet Gynecol 179:1479–1484, 1998).

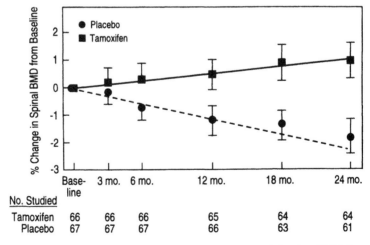

Fig. 7-7. Change in mean (± SE) lumbar spine bone mineral density (BMD) in women with breast cancer given tamoxifen or placebo for 2 years. (Adapted from N Engl J Med 326:854, 1992. Copyright © 1992 Massachusetts Medical Society. All rights reserved.)

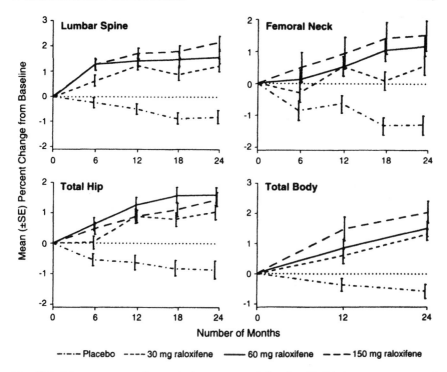

Fig. 7-8. Mean percent change in bone mineral density (BMD) in postmenopasual women receiving raloxifene or placebo for 2 years. (Adapted from N Engl J Med:1644, 1997. Copyright © 1997 Massachusetts Medical Society. All rights reserved.)

prevention, but the demonstration of prevention of bone loss in animal models, with no toxic effects, ultimately led to its development as an agent for prevention of osteoporosis. The drug, which received FDA approval in the United States in 1998, prevents bone loss in postmenopausal women (Fig. 7-8). Two years of therapy with raloxifene produces a modest, but significant, increase in BMD in the spine, hip, and total body, of the order of 2–3% over that observed in placebo-treated individuals. These changes in BMD are associated with a decrease in the risk of vertebral fracture by approximately 45% at the marketed dose of 60 mg/day, with little if any apparent effect on peripheral fractures. Raloxifene has also been shown to produce effects on blood lipids that are somewhat similar to those of estrogens. Total and LDL cholesterol are lowered. Total HDL does not change, although HDL_2 increases. The increment in HDL_2 is approximately 50% that seen with estrogen treatment. Unlike estrogen, raloxifene does not increase blood triglycerides. These combined effects suggest that raloxifene should produce a favorable effect on cardiovascular disease, although disease outcome data in humans are not yet available for analyses. Currently, animal data are conflicting, with no evidence for a positive effect of raloxifene in the monkey

**TABLE 7-5. Risk of Pulmonary Embolus in Estrogen Users
Nurses Health Study 1976–1992**

Treatment Group	Cases	Person Years	Relative Risk (95% CI)	
			Adjusted for Age and Smoking	Adjusted for Risk Factors
Postmenopausal hormone use (postmenopausal women)				
Never	27	320,339	1.0	1.0
Current	22	155,669	1.8 (1.0-3.2)	2.1 (1.2-3.8)
Past	19	157,809	1.4 (0.8-2.4)	1.3 (0.7-2.4)
Oral contraceptive use				
Never	76	829,240	1.0	1.0
Current	5	21,857	2.1 (0.7-6.1)	2.2 (0.8-5.9)
Past	42	709,469	0.8 (0.5-1.1)	0.8 (0.5-1.2)

Grodstein *et al:* Lancet 348:983–987, 1996. © by The Lancet Ltd.

model of altheroma, while positive effects have been observed in rabbits receiving raloxifene, with reduction of arterial wall cholesterol accumulation. As has been demonstrated in observational studies, and one clinical trial for hormonal replacement therapy, raloxifene produces an increase in venous thrombosis comparable to that observed for estrogen (Table 7-5).

Unlike both estrogen and tamoxifen, raloxifene used for 2 years or more, does not stimulate the endometrium, but unlike estrogen may increase the occurrence of hot flashes in those females predisposed to these symptoms (6% greater than placebo). A most gratifying observation is that raloxifene does produce rather dramatic effects on the occurrence of breast cancer, with a 76% reduction in the appearance of new cancers in healthy postmenopausal women over a 3-year exposure period. Currently, the U.S. National Cancer Institute is sponsoring a head-to-head trial of tamoxifen and raloxifene in preventing breast cancer among 22,000 women in 400 medical centers in the United States and Canada.

Although technically a second generation SERM, raloxifene seems likely to be the first in a long line of agents tailored to produce the beneficial effects of estrogen without the perceived negative effects. At present, raloxifene is a useful agent for prevention of osteoporosis for use in postmenopausal women who refuse estrogen therapy categorically and those who cannot or will not comply to treatment regimens using progesterone.

SUGGESTED READING

Estrogens

Anderson FH, Francis RM, Selby PL, Cooper C: Editorial: Sex hormones and osteoporosis in men. Calcif Tissue Int 62:185–188, 1998.

Barrett-Connor E, Stuenkel CA: Guest Editorial: Anticipating HERS: Questions from the heart and estrogen–progestin replacement study. J Women's Health 7:395–397.

Grady D, Sawaya G: Postmenopausal hormone therapy increases risk of deep vein thrombosis and pulmonary embolism. Am J Med 105:41–43, 1998.

Greenspan SL, Myers ER, Kiel DP, Parker RA, Hayes WC, Resnick NM: Fall direction, bone mineral density, and function: Risk factors for hip fracture in frail nursing home elderly. Excerpta Medica 104:539–545, 1998.

Hulley S, Grady D, Bush T, Furberg C, Herrington D, Riggs B, Vittinghoff E: Randomized trial of estrogen plus progestin for secondary prevention of coronary heart disease in postmenopausal women. JAMA 280:605–613, 1998.

Ikegami A, Inoue S, Hosoi T, Mizuno Y, Nakamura T, Ouchi Y, Orimo H: Immunohistochemical detection and Northern blot analysis of estrogen receptor in osteoblastic cells. J Bone Miner Res 8:1103–1109, 1993.

Kado DM, Browner WS, Palermo L, Nevitt MC, Genant HK, Cummings SR: Vertebral fractures and mortality in older women. A prospective study. Arch Intern Med 159:1215–1220, 1999.

Keating NL, Cleary PD, Rossi AS, Zaslavsky AM, Ayanian JZ: Use of hormone replacement therapy for postmenopausal women in the United States. Ann Intern Med 130:545–553, 1999.

Khosla S, Atkinson EJ, Melton LJ III, Rigss BL: Effects of age and estrogen status on serum parathyroid hormone levels and biochemical markers of bone turnover in women: A population-based study. J Clin Endocrinol Metab 82:1522–1527, 1997.

Komulainen M, Kroger H, Tuppurainen MT, Heikknen AM, Alhava E, Honkanen R, Jurvelin J, Saarikoski S: Prevention of femoral and lumbar bone loss with hormone replacement therapy and vitamin D3 in early postmenopausal women: A population-based 5-year randomized trial. J Clin Endocrinol Metab 84:546–552, 1999.

LeBoff MS, Kohlmeier L, Hurwitz S, Franklin J, Wright J, Glowacki J: Occult vitamin D deficiency in postmenopausal U.S. women with acute hip fracture. JAMA 281:1505–1511, 1999.

Legault C, Espeland MA, Wasilauskas CH, Bush TL, Trabal J, Judd HL, Johnson SR, Greendale GA: Agreement in assessing endometrial pathology: The postmenopausal estrogen/progestin interventions (PEPI) trial. J Women's Health 7:435–442, 1998.

Lindsay R: The role of estrogen in the prevention of osteoporosis. Endocrinol Metab Clin North America 27:399–409, 1998.

Maricic M: Early prevention vs. late treatment for osteoporosis. Arch Intern Med 157:2545–2546, 1997.

Mendelsoh ME, Karas RH: The protective effects of estrogen on the cardiovascular system. Mech Dis 340:1801–1811, 1999.

Michaelsson K, Baron JA, Johnell O, Persson I, Ljunghall S: Variation in the efficacy of hormone replacement therapy in the prevention of hip fracture. Osteoporosis Int 8:540–546, 1998.

Nguyen TV, Jones G, Sambrook PH, White CP, Kelly PJ, Eisman JA: Effects of estrogen exposure and reproductive factors on bone mineral density and osteoporotic fractures. J Clin Endocrinol Metab 80:2709–2714, 1995.

Nieves JW, Komar L, Cosman F, Lindsay R: Calcium potentiates the effect of estrogen and calcitonin on bone mass: Review and analysis. Am J Clin Nutr 67:18–24, 1998.

Orwoll ES, Nelson HD: Does estrogen adequately protect postmenopausal women against osteoporosis: An iconoclastic perspective. J Clin Endocrinol Metab 84: 1872–1874, 1999.

Payne JB, Reinhardt RA, Nummikoski PV, Patil KD: Longitudinal alveolar bone loss in postmenopausal osteoporotic/osteopenic women. Osteoporosis Int 10:34–40, 1999.

Phillips SK, Rook KM, Siddle NC, Bruce SA, Woledge RC: Muscle weakness in women occurs at an earlier age than in men, but strength is preserved by hormone replacement therapy. Clin Sci 84:95–98, 1993.

Recker RR, Davies KM, Dowd RM, Heaney RP: The effect of low-dose continuous estrogen and progesterone therapy with calcium and vitamin D on bone in elderly women. A randomized, controlled trial. Ann Intern Med 130:897–904, 1999.

Reginster JV, Sarlet N, Deroisy R, Albert A, Gaspard U, Franchimont P: Minimal levels of serum estradiol prevent postmenopasual bone loss. Calcif Tissue Int 51:340–343, 1992.

Santoro NF, Col NF, Eckman MH, Wong JB, Pauker SG, Cauley JA, Zmuda J, Crawford S, Johannes CB, Rossouw JE, Bairey Merz CN: Hormone replacement therapy—Where are we going? J Clin Endocrinol Metab 84:1798–1802, 1999.

SERM Drugs

Balfour JA, Coa KL: Raloxifene. Drug Aging 12:335–343, 1998.

Barrett-Connor E, Wenger NK, Grady D, Mosca L, Collins P, Kornitzer M, Cox DA, Moscarelli E, Anderson PW: Hormone and nonhormone therapy for the maintenance of postmenopausal health: The need for randomized controlled trials of estrogen and raloxifene. J Women's Health 7:839–847, 1998.

Brzozowski AM, Pike ACW, Dauter Z, Hubbard RE, Bonn T, Engstrom O, Ohman L, Greene GL, Gustafsson JA, Carlquist M: Molecular basis of agonism and antagonism in the oestrogen receptor. Nature (London) 389:753–758, 1997.

Clarkson TB, Anthony MS, Jerome CP: Lack of effect of raloxifene on coronary artery atherosclerosis of postmenopausal monkeys. J Clin Endocrinol Metab 83:721–726, 1998.

Cosman F, Lindsay R: Selective estrogen receptor modulators: Clinical spectrum. Endocr Rev 20:418–434, 1999.

Cummings SR, Eckert S, Krueger KA, Crady D, Powles TJ, Cauley JA, Norton L, Nickelsen T, Bjarnason NH, Morrow M, Lippman ME, Black D, Clusman JE, Costa A, Jordan VC: The effect of raloxifene on risk of breast cancer in postmenopausal women. Results from the MORE randomized trial. JAMA 281:2189–2197, 1999.

Delmas PD, Bjarnason NH, Mitlak BH, Ravoux AC, Shah AS, Huster WJ, Draper M, Christiansen C: Effects of raloxifene on bone mineral density, serum cholesterol concentrations, and uterine endometrium in postmenopausal women. N Engl J Med 337:1641–1647, 1997.

Goldstein SR: Selective estrogen receptor modulators: A new category of therapeutic agents for extending the health of postmenopausal women. Am J Obstet Gynecol 179:1479–1484, 1998.

Grey AB, Stapleton JP, Evans MC, Tatnell MA, Ames RW, Reid IR: The effect of the antiestrogen tamoxifen on bone mineral density in normal late postmenopausal women. Am J Med 99:636–641, 1995.

Heaney RP, Draper MW: Raloxifene and estrogen: Comparative bone-remodeling kinetics. J Clin Endocrinol Metab 82:3425–3429, 1997.

Jordan VC: Designer estrogens. These compounds—also called SERMs—have evolved from mere laboratory curiosities into drugs that hold promise for preventing several major disorders in women. Scientific American 60–67, October, 1998.

Lindsay R, Cosman F: Skeletal effects of estrogen analogs. Osteoporosis Int 1:S40–S42, 1997.

Lufkin EG, Whitaker MD, Kickelsen T, Argueta R, Caplan RH, Knickerbocker RK, Riggs BL: Treatment of established postmenopausal osteoporosis with Raloxifene: A randomized trial. J Bone Miner Res 13:1747–1754, 1998.

Mitlak BH, Cohen FJ: Selective estrogen receptor modulators. A look ahead. Drugs 57:653–663, 1999.

Sadovsky Y, Adler S: Editorial: Selective modulation of estrogen receptor action. J Clin Endocrinol Metab 83:3–5, 1998.

Tremblay A, Tremblay GB, Labrie C, Labrie F, Giguere V: EM-800, a novel antiestrogen, acts as a pure antagonist of the transcriptional functions of estrogen receptors α and β. Endocrinology (Baltimore) 139:111–118, 1998.

Walsh BW, Kuller LH, Wild RA, Paul S, Farmer M, Lawrence JB, Shah AS, Anderson PW: Effects of Raloxifene on serum lipids and coagulation factors in healthy postmenopausal women. JAMA 279:1445–1451, 1998.

Ward RL, Morgan G, Dalley D, Kelly PJ: Tamoxifen reduces bone turnover and prevents lumbar spine and proximal femoral bone loss in early postmenopausal women. Bone Miner 22:87–94, 1993.

Yaffe K, Sawaya G, Lieberburg I, Grady D: Estrogen therapy in postmenopausal women: Effects on cognitive function and dementia. JAMA 279:688–695, 1998.

8 Bisphosphonate Treatment for Osteoporosis

Nelson B. Watts

INTRODUCTION

Bisphosphonates (once called diphosphonates) have a chemical structure similar to pyrophosphates. Pyrophosphates consist of two phosphonic acids joined to an oxygen [phosphorus–oxygen–phosphorus (P — O — P) structure]; bisphosphonates have a phosphorus–carbon–phosphorus (P — C — P) structure (Fig. 8-1). The P — O — P bonds are easily cleaved by pyrophosphatases; the P — C — P structure is essentially impervious to chemical and enzymatic breakdown. The two phosphonic acids cause bisphosphonates to be adsorbed onto the surface of hydroxyapatite crystals in bone, primarily at sites of active bone remodeling.

The first bisphosphonates were synthesized over 100 years ago. Initially, they were used in industry (and still are used) as antiscaling and anticorrosive agents in washing powders and water and oil brines to prevent the deposition of calcium carbonate scale. The first recorded medical use was in the 1960s. Bisphosphonates have potential applications for a variety of diagnostic and therapeutic purposes. They are used as carriers for radioactive tracers for imaging in nuclear bone scans. Along with drugs such as estrogen, selective estrogen-receptor modulators (SERMs), and calcitonin, bisphosphonates alter bone remodeling by reducing bone resorption and are considered to be "antiresorptive" agents. In addition to being used for the prevention and treatment of osteoporosis due to various etiologies, bisphosphonates have been used to treat myositis ossificans progressiva; fibrous dysplasia of bone; osteogenesis imperfecta; heterotopic ossification; Paget's disease of bone; hypercalcemia due to immobilization, malignancy, and

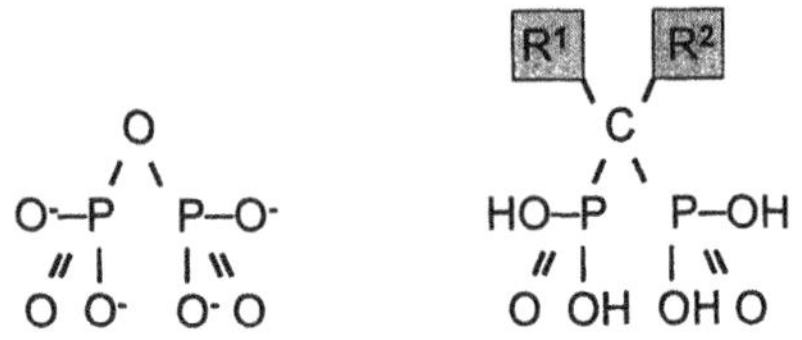

Fig. 8-1. Structures of pyrophosphate and bisphosphonates. The P — O — P bonds of pyrophosphates are readily degraded by ubiquitous enzymes, pyrophosphatases; the P — C — P bonds of bisphosphonates are essentially impervious to enzymatic degradation. The bisphosphonate side chains, R^1 and R^2, can be substituted to alter affinity for bone and antiresorptive potency, respectively.

other causes; destructive arthropathy (Charcot joints); reflex sympathetic dystrophy; skeletal involvement with metastatic cancer or multiple myeloma; and to reduce the risk of bone metastases from cancer. They appear to have potential benefits in any condition involving increased bone remodeling.

As shown in Fig. 8-1, bisphosphonates have two side chains, R^1 and R^2. Altering the side chains changes the potency and side effect profile of the compounds (Table 8-1). *In vitro,* the antiresorptive properties increase at least 100-fold between generations, but *in vivo,* the difference is approximately 10-fold.

MECHANISMS OF ACTION

Bisphosphonates bind to bone surfaces and are released locally in the acid environment created by osteoclasts. Once they enter the osteoclast they reduce the production of acid and enzymes beneath the ruffled border of

TABLE 8-1. Structures of Some Bisphosphonates in Clinical Use

First generation (R^2 is short alkyl group or halogen)		
Compound	R^1	R^2
Etidronate	OH	CH_3
Clodronate	Cl	Cl
Second generation (R^2 has amino-terminal group)		
Compound	R^1	R^2
Pamidronate	OH	$CH_2CH_2NH_2$
Alendronate	OH	$CH_2CH_2CH_2NH_2$
Third generation (R^2 is cyclic side chain)		
Compound	R^1	R^2
Risedronate	OH	CH_2-3-pyridinyl
Ibandronate	OH	$CH_2CH_2N(CH_3)CH_2CH_2CH_2CH_2CH_3$

the osteoclast, which decreases the ability of the osteoclast to resorb bone. Bisphosphonates also may reduce the activation of osteoclast precursors, the differentiation of precursor cells into mature osteoclasts, chemotaxis, and attachment of osteoclasts to bone. Some of the differences in antiresorptive potencies of various bisphosphonates are due in part to differing actions at early steps in the remodeling process. An intriguing aspect of bisphosphonate action is their ability to increase apoptosis (programmed cell death) of osteoclasts. Clodronate and etidronate do this by being incorporated into nonmetabolizable analogs of ATP; alendronate, risedronate, and other nitrogen-containing bisphosphonates interfere with the mevalonate pathway and protein prenylation.

Bisphosphonates reduce activation frequency (the rate at which new bone remodeling units are formed). They also reduce the depth of resorption and produce a positive bone balance at individual remodeling units. This reduction in resorption depth protects against trabecular perforation, maintains or improves bone quality, and reduces the risk for future fracture. The positive bone balance at each remodeling unit explains the continued increase of bone mass with long-term use.

ALENDRONATE

Alendronate (Fosamax) is currently (April 1999) the only bisphosphonate approved by the United States Food and Drug Administration (FDA) for use in osteoporosis. Alendronate at 5 mg daily is approved for prevention of bone loss in recently menopausal women, and alendronate at 10 mg daily is approved for treatment of established osteoporosis.

The Early Postmenopausal Intervention Cohort (EPIC) is an ongoing study to assess the effect of alendronate for prevention of the accelerated phase of bone loss that occurs in early menopause. In preliminary results of what is planned to be a 6-year study in which 1609 women were enrolled (average age early 50s and about 2 years postmenopause), Hosking et al. (1998) showed that the 5 mg of alendronate daily prevented bone loss at the spine (Fig. 8-2) and hip.

Two large placebo-controlled, double-blind Phase III studies were conducted (two protocols with identical study design), one arm at 18 centers in the United States and the other at 19 multinational centers. These centers recruited 994 women with postmenopausal osteoporosis (spinal bone density ≥2.5 SD below peak bone mass) who were randomly assigned to one of four groups: placebo, alendronate 5 mg daily for 3 years, alendronate 10 mg daily for 3 years, and alendronate 20 mg daily (changed to 5 mg daily for the third year). Particularly apparent in the U.S. cohort, the effect on bone mass appeared maximal with 10 mg alendronate daily (Fig. 8-3), and this effect did not appear to plateau after 3 years of treatment (average gain in spine

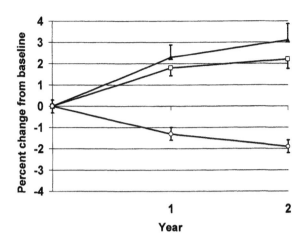

Fig. 8-2. Mean percent change (± SE) in spinal bone mineral density as measured by dual-energy X-ray absorptiometry in the placebo (circles), 2.5 mg (squares), and 5 mg (triangles) alendronate treatment groups of the Early Postmenopausal Intervention Cohort (EPIC) study. (After data from Hosking D, Chilvers CED, Christiansen C, Ravn P, Wasnich R, Ross P, McClung M, Blaske A, Thompson D, Daley M, Yates AJ: Prevention of bone loss with alendronate in postmenopausal women under 60 years of age. Early Postmenopausal Intervention Cohort Study Group. N Engl J Med 338:485–492, 1998. Copyright 1998 Massachusetts Medical Society. All rights reserved.)

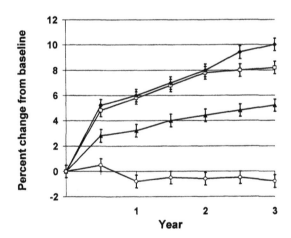

Fig. 8-3. Mean percent change (± SE) in spinal bone mineral density as measured by dual-energy X-ray absorptiometry in the placebo (circles), 5 mg (triangles), 10 mg (closed diamonds), and 20/5 mg (squares) alendronate treatment groups of the U.S. Phase III Alendronate Study in women with established postmenopausal osteoporosis. (Reprinted from Am J Med 101. Tucci R, Tonino RP, Emkey RD, *et al:* Effect of three years of oral alendronate treatment in postmenopausal women with osteoporosis, 488–501. Copyright 1996, with permission from Excerpta Medica Inc.)

bone mineral density, ~6% at 1 year, a further ~2% in year 2, and ~2% more in year 3, for a total of almost 10% increase after 3 years).

The Phase III studies of alendronate were not powered to show an effect on fractures. However, pooling of data from all of the alendronate groups from both U.S. and multinational centers showed a 48% reduction in fractures compared with placebo (3.2 versus 6.2%). To fully assess the impact of alendronate therapy on fractures, the Fracture Intervention Trial (FIT) was undertaken, recruiting women age 55–80 with low femoral neck bone mineral density (BMD) (≥2.5 SD below peak bone mass) who were randomized to receive either placebo or alendronate. In a group of over 2000 women at high risk of fracture, the study was planned for 3 years but was terminated early because the reduction in fracture risk was already significant (Fig. 8-4). The reduction in fracture risk was 55% for clinically apparent vertebral fracture, 51% for hip fracture, and 48% for wrist fracture. In an additional 4434 women with low bone mass but no fracture on enrollment to the study, a fracture benefit was shown after 4 years. Alendronate has also been shown to be effective for treatment and prevention of glucocorticoid-induced bone loss.

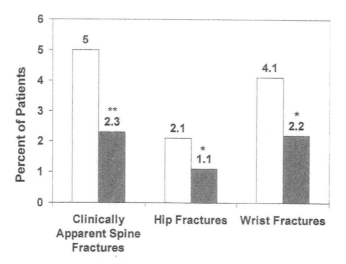

Fig. 8-4. Percent of patients in the control group (open bars) and alendronate group (shaded bars) in Arm 1 of the Fracture Intervention Trial (FIT) having new fractures during the course of the study. **$p < .001$, *$p < .05$ between groups. (From Black DM, Cummings SR, Karpf DB, Cauley JA, Thompson DE, Nevitt MC, Bauer DC, Genant HK, Haskell WL, Marcus R, Ott SM, Torner JC, Quandt SA, Reiss TF, Ensrud KE: Randomised trial of effect of alendronate on risk of fracture in women with existing vertebral fractures. Fracture Intervention Trial Research Group. Lancet 348:1535–1541, 1996, used with permission).

OTHER BISPHOSPHONATES

Several other bisphosphonates are approved by the FDA for nonosteoporosis indications (e.g., Paget's disease, hypercalcemia) and therefore available in the United States. These include etidronate, tiludronate, pamidronate (available in the United States as an intravenous infusion, and in Europe as an oral preparation), and risedronate. Other bisphosphonates, such as clodronate, olpadronate, and incandronate, are available in other countries. Still others, such as ibandronate and zoledronate, are in clinical development.

Etidronate

Etidronate (Didronel, EHDP) was the first bisphosphonate in clinical use. Oral etidronate is approved by the FDA for treatment of Paget's disease of bone and heterotopic ossification, and an intravenous form of the drug is approved for the treatment of hypercalcemia of malignancy. Although etidronate is not approved in the United States for treatment of osteoporosis, it has been approved in all other countries (22) that have pharmaceutical regulatory agencies.

Because continuous etidronate treatment is known to impair mineralization of new bone, an intermittent cyclical regimen is used to treat osteoporosis. A typical regimen is to give 400 mg of oral etidronate (5–10 mg/kg/day) once daily for 14 days and to repeat the 2-week course of treatment approximately every 3 months. The effectiveness of intermittent cyclical etidronate treatment for postmenopausal osteoporosis was confirmed by two prospective, randomized, controlled trials (one from Denmark and the other from the United States) which showed that intermittent cyclical therapy with etidronate (plus calcium) resulted in significant increases in spinal bone mass.

In the Danish study, which involved 66 women with severe osteoporosis, rates of vertebral fractures were significantly lower in the treated patients compared with controls. The U.S. multicenter study included 423 women, most with mild osteoporosis. The rate of new vertebral fractures was low in this population because of the mild degree of osteoporosis. Nevertheless, during the 2 years of blinded treatment, the rate of new vertebral fractures was significantly lower by 50% in patients who received etidronate compared with those who did not (29.5 fractures per 1000 patient years compared with 62.9 fractures per 1000 patient years, respectively). Although these results have been viewed as generally positive, this study has been criticized because of the low fracture rate.

Patients from the U.S. study were continued on blinded therapy for a third year and then changed to open label therapy for an additional 2 years, then rerandomized to continue treatment or change to placebo for a further 2 years. After 3 years of blinded treatment, bone mineral density increased at all hip sites in patients treated with etidronate. In both groups, rates of

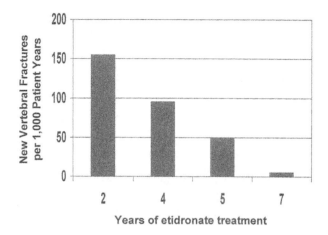

Years of etidronate treatment

Fig. 8-5. Rate of new vertebral fractures per 1000 patient years as a function of years of treatment with intermittent cyclical etidronate. (Reprinted from Am J Med 103; Miller PD, Watts NB, Licata AA, Harris ST, Genant HK, Wasnich RD, Ross PD, Jackson RD, Hoseyni MS, Schoenfeld SL, Valent DJ, Chesnut CHI: Cyclical etidronate in the treatment of postmenopausal osteoporosis: Efficacy and safety after 7 years of treatment, 468–476. Copyright 1997, with permission from Excerpta Medica Inc.)

vertebral fractures remained lower than in the initial 3 years of observation in the control group. In years 6 and 7, spinal bone density increased significantly in the patients who continued treatment and remained stable for 2 years of observation in the patients who were withdrawn after 2 years and 5 years of treatment. The incidence of new vertebral fractures was very low in years 6 and 7 and correlated with the duration of treatment (Fig. 8-5). Only one patient who had been on treatment for 7 years had a new fracture during the last phase of the study. Etidronate has also been shown to prevent bone loss in recently menopausal women and to be effective for treatment and prevention of corticosteroid-induced osteoporosis.

Pamidronate

Pamidronate (Aredia, also known as APD) has been used to treat hypercalcemia of malignancy and Paget's disease of bone. Oral therapy with 150 to 300 mg pamidronate daily has been shown to improve bone density in the spine. However, a large U.S. Phase III study of oral pamidronate was terminated because of the frequent occurrence of esophageal side effects. The main role for pamidronate in management of osteoporosis patients in the United States is given by intravenous infusion to patients who cannot tolerate oral bisphosphonates. For this purpose, a regimen of 30 mg (infused over 1 to 2 h) given every third month has been used with some reports of improved bone density. Both oral and intravenous pamidronate appear to be effective for treatment of corticosteroid-induced osteoporosis.

Intravenous pamidronate has been shown to reduce morbidity and mortality in patients with multiple myeloma and to reduce skeletal complications in patients with breast cancer who have lytic bone metastases.

Clodronate

Clodronate is not available in the United States. In Europe, it has been used both orally and intravenously to treat osteoporosis. An intermittent intravenous regimen (200 mg infused every 3 weeks), an oral cyclical regimen (400 mg daily for 25 days, then 60 days off), and continuous oral therapy (400 mg daily) all resulted in spinal bone mineral density significantly higher compared with controls. A higher dose regimen of clodronate, 1600 mg daily, has been show to reduce new metastases in breast cancer patients.

Tiludronate

Tiludronate (Skelid) is approved in the United States for treatment of Paget's disease. A large Phase III trial of tiludronate for treatment of osteoporosis was terminated because of apparent lack of effect, possibly because the dose being studied was too low.

Risedronate

Risedronate (Actonel) is approved in the United States for treatment of Paget's disease. Approval for osteoporosis is pending with the FDA. Large-scale trials for treatment and prevention of postmenopausal osteoporosis and corticosteroid-induced osteoporosis have been completed and should soon be published.

ABSORPTION AND RETENTION

Bisphosphonates are poorly absorbed after oral administration. Typically, less than 5% of an oral dose is absorbed. Absorption is significantly reduced or eliminated if the drug is taken with calcium, other divalent cations, or with foods or beverages other than water. With some compounds, bioavailability remains negligible even 2 h after a meal. Bisphosphonates should be taken with water (coffee or orange juice may reduce the absorption by 50%). Because of the interference of food with absorption, they should be taken first thing in the morning, after an overnight fast, with nothing by mouth for at least 30 min (and possibly longer). After an appropriate interval (but not before), food, medications, calcium, etc. may be taken.

About 50% of the absorbed bisphosphonate binds to bone surfaces within 12 to 24 h. After the drug exerts its effect, the remainder becomes buried in bone, where it is retained for months or years but is no longer active. Bisphosphonates are not metabolized systemically; drug which does not bind to skeletal sites, is excreted unchanged in the urine. Because of the renal route of elimination, bisphosphonates should be given with caution or not at all to patients with renal insufficiency.

SIDE EFFECTS, TOXICITY

Bisphosphonates are safe and generally well tolerated. Continuous treatment with etidronate causes impaired mineralization of bone; the intermittent cyclical regimen used for treatment of osteoporosis avoids this problem. Gastrointestinal complaints are the most common side effects—nausea and diarrhea with etidronate and clodronate, and upper gastrointestinal side effects (nausea, dyspepsia, inflammation or ulcers of the esophagus, stomach, and duodenum) are seen with oral administration of aminobisphosphonates (pamidronate and alendronate), rarely resulting in erosive esophagitis or bleeding. Perhaps 10% of patients who try alendronate cannot continue to take it. Serious reactions are infrequent, approximately 1:10,000. To minimize esophageal irritation, alendronate should be taken with 6 to 8 ounces of water (to be certain that the tablet passes through the esophagus and into the stomach), and the patient must remain upright (seated or standing) until after eating, to avoid reflux of drug into the esophagus. Alendronate should not be given to patients who cannot remain upright, or to patients who have active upper gastrointestinal symptoms, or who have delayed esophageal emptying (e.g., strictures, achalasia, or severe dysmotility), and it should be discontinued if such problems develop during its use (e.g., therapy should be stopped if the patient becomes temporarily bedfast or develops difficulty swallowing, retrosternal pain, or new or increased heartburn).

Acute-phase reactions (fever and lymphopenia) occur in 10–20% of patients given their first intravenous infusion of pamidronate (and possibly with other intravenous bisphosphonates) but may not recur with repeated administration. Hypocalcemia may also occur with rapid parenteral administration of bisphosphonates, but is infrequent and usually mild. Acute renal failure has been seen with rapid intravenous infusions of etidronate and clodronate, a problem that should not occur with appropriate infusion rates. Several cases of leukemia were reported in early trials with clodronate, although clodronate was not thought to be causally related. Clodronate, pamidronate, and tiludronate have been associated with severe toxic skin reactions. Eye complications (uveitis, scleritis, episcleritis, and conjunctivitis) have been seen with pamidronate, with a frequency of about 1:1000.

FUTURE DIRECTIONS

A third-generation bisphosphonate, ibandronate, is in the late stages of Phase III trials with a regimen of intravenous injection every third month. Intermittent oral dosing (once or twice weekly) is being investigated with some established bisphosphonates, both to improve patient acceptance and possibly to reduce gastrointestinal side effects.

COMBINATION THERAPY (BISPHOSPHONATES PLUS OTHER ANTIRESORPTIVES)

There has been concern that combining two or more antiresorptive agents (such as estrogen plus a bisphosphonate) might oversuppress bone remodeling and lead to "frozen bone." There is no evidence that this occurs, and there is some evidence that combining bisphosphonates with estrogen or adding a bisphosphonate to estrogen will result in greater increases in bone mass than either given alone. Whether the additional gains in bone mass provide further reduction in fractures is not known. Certainly, it appears to be safe to use bisphosphonates with estrogen. Theoretically, bisphosphonates could also be used in combination with raloxifene or calcitonin, but there are no studies addressing this.

SUMMARY

Bisphosphonates, compounds that share a $P-C-P$ structure, bind avidly to bone at sites of active remodeling. They inhibit osteoclast recruitment, reduce osteoclast activity, and accelerate apoptosis. Alendronate is the only bisphosphonate currently approved by the U.S. FDA. Etidronate, which is given in an intermittent cyclic regimen, is not approved by the FDA for osteoporosis but is approved for this indication in other countries and is available in the United States, and is a good choice for patients who need a bisphosphonate but cannot take alendronate. Pamidronate, given by intravenous infusion, is an alternative for patients who cannot take oral bisphosphonates.

Bisphosphonates are generally well tolerated. They appear to be effective for prevention and treatment of postmenopausal osteoporosis, corticosteroid-induced osteoporosis, and other forms of bone loss. These agents have an important role in prevention and treatment of osteoporosis; however, more research is needed regarding optimal doses and regimens (continuous versus intermittent), comparisons with other agents, and use in combination with other agents.

SUGGESTED READING

Adachi JD, Bensen WG, Brown J, Hanley D, Hodsman A, Josse R, Kendler, DL, Lentle B, Olszynski W, Ste-Marie LG, Tenenhouse A, Chines AA: Intermittent etidronate therapy to prevent corticosteroid-induced osteoporosis. N Engl J Med 337: 382–387, 1997.

Black DM, Cummings SR, Karpf DB, Cauley JA, Thompson DE, Nevitt MC, Bauer DC, Genant HK, Haskell WL, Marcus R, Ott SM, Torner JC, Quandt, SA, Reiss TF, Ensrud KE: Randomised trial of effect of alendronate on risk of fracture in women with existing vertebral fractures. Fracture Intervention Trial Research Group. Lancet 348:1535–1541, 1996.

Cummings SR, Black MD, Thompson DE, Applegate WB, Barrett-Connor E, Musliner TA, Palermo L, Prineas R, Rubin SM, Scott JC, Vogt T, Wallace R, Yates AJ, LaCroix AZ for the Fracture Intervention Trial Research Group: JAMA 280:2077–2082, 1998.

Diel IJ, Solomayer E-F, Costa SD, Gollan C, Goerner R, Wallwiener D, Kaufmann M, Bastert G: Reductions in new metastases in breast cancer with adjuvant clodronate treatment. N Engl J Med 339:357–363, 1998.

Fleisch H: Bisphosphonates: Mechanisms of action. Endocr Rev 19:80–100, 1998.

Hortobagyi GN, Theriault RL, Porter L, Blayney D, Lipton A, Sinoff C, Wheeler H, Simeone JF, Seaman J, Knight RD, Heffernan M, Reitsma DJ: Efficacy of pamidronate in reducing skeletal complications in patients with breast cancer and lytic bone metastases. N Engl J Med 335:1785–1791, 1996.

Hosking D, Chilvers CED, Christiansen C, Ravn P, Wasnich R, Ross P, McClung M, Balske A, Thompson D, Daley M, Yates AJ: Prevention of bone loss with alendronate in postmenopausal women under 60 years of age. Early Postmenopausal Intervention Cohort Study Group. N Engl J Med 338:485–492, 1998.

Liberman UA, Weiss SR, Broll J, Minne HW, Quan H, Bell NH, Rodriguez-Portales J, Downs RW Jr, Dequeker J, Favus M: Effect of oral alendronate on bone mineral density and the incidence of fractures in postmenopausal osteoporosis. N Engl J Med 333:1437–1443, 1995.

Meunier PJ, Confavreux E, Tuoinen J, Harduoin C, Delmas PD, Balena R: Prevention of early postmenopausal bone loss with cyclical etidronate therapy (a double-blind, placebo-controlled study and 1-year follow-up. J Clin Endocrinol Metab 82:2784–2791, 1997.

Miller PD, Watts NB, Licata AA, Harris ST, Genant HK, Wasnich RD, Ross PD, Jackson RD, Hoseyni MS, Schoenfeld SL, Valent DJ, Chesnut CHI: Cyclical etidronate in the treatment of postmenopausal osteoporosis: Efficacy and safety after 7 years of treatment. Am J Med 103:468–476, 1997.

Saag KG, Emkey R, Schnitzer TJ, Brown JP, Hawkins F, Goemaere S, Thamsborg G, Liberman UA, Delmas PD, Malice M-P, Czachur M, Daifotis AG for the

Glucocortoid-Induced Osteoporosis Intervention Study Group: Alendronate for the prevention and treatment of glucocorticoid-induced osteoporosis. N Engl J Med 339:292–299, 1998.

Stock JL, Bell NH, Chesnutt CH III, Ensrud KE, Genant HK, Harris ST, McClung MR, Singer FR, Yood RA, Pryor-Tillotson S, Wei L, Santora AC III: Increments in bone mineral density of the lumbar spine and hip and suppression of bone turnover are maintained after discontinuation of alendronate in postmenopausal women. Am J Med 103:291–297, 1997.

Thiebaud D, Burckhardt P, Melchior J, Eckert P, Jacquet AF, Schnyder P, Gobelet C: Two year effectiveness of intravenous pamidronate (APD) versus oral fluoride for osteoporosis occurring in the menopause. Osteoporosis Int 4:76–83, 1994.

Thiebaud D, Burckhardt P, Kriegbaum H, Huss H, Mulder H, Juttmann JR, Schoter KH: Three monthly intravenous injections of ibandronate in the treatment of post-menopausal osteoporosis. Am J Med 103:298–307, 1997.

Tucci JR, Tonino, RP, Emkey RD *et al:* Effect of three years of oral alendronate treat-ment in postmenopausal women with osteoporosis. Am J Med 101:488–501, 1996.

Watts NB: Treatment of osteoporosis with bisphosphonates. Endocrinol Metabol Clin North Am 27:419–439, 1998.

Wimalawansa SJ: Combined therapy with estrogen and etidronate has an additive effect on bone mineral density in the hip and vertebrae: Four-year randomized study. Am J Med 99:36–42.

Wimalawansa SJ: A four-year randomized controlled trial of hormone replacement and bisphosphonate, alone or in combination, in women with postmenopausal osteoporosis. Am J Med 104:219–226, 1998.

9   Calcitonin Treatment in Postmenopausal Osteoporosis

Stuart L. Silverman

INTRODUCTION

In 1961, it was observed that a hypocalcemic factor was released by the thyroid–parathyroid glands in response to perfusion with blood high in calcium. This factor, which modulated the "tone" of calcium in extracellular fluids and was named calcitonin, was subsequently shown to be produced by the parafollicular "C" cells of the thyroid gland. It was later demonstrated that the calcitonin gene peptide superfamily consists of calcitonin, calcitonin gene-related peptide, amylin, and adrenomedullin. These structurally related polypeptides are characterized by a six- or seven-amino acid ring structure linked by a disulfide bridge and an amidated C terminus. A portion of the β chain of insulin is strongly homologous to these four polypeptides, suggesting a possible historical relationship to the insulin gene superfamily. Calcitonins are 32-amino acid polypeptide hormones with a 1–7 amino-terminal disulfide bridge, a glycine at residue 28, and a carboxyl-terminal proline amide residue. There is no biologically active fragment. Calcitonins are found in a number of animal species, and the majority of studies designed to stabilize bone mass in humans have been performed with salmon, eel, and human calcitonins. In this regard, salmon and eel calcitonins are the most potent forms per milligram, with 50–100 times the potency of other mammalian forms of the hormone. Other tissue sources of calcitonin include the pituitary and neuroendocrine cells. Malignant transformation can occur in both ectopic and normal cells which produce calcitonin, and the peptide then becomes a tumor marker. The best examples of this process are medullary carcinoma of the thyroid and small cell lung cancer.

Calcitonin inhibits bone resorption by interfering with osteoclast activity. After exposure to calcitonin, osteoclasts undergo flattening of their metabolically active ruffled border and withdraw from sites of bone resorption. Calcitonin prevents hypercalcemia following calcium rich meals and protects calcium stores during periods of calcium stress such as pregnancy, lactation, and low dietary calcium intake. Despite these biological responses, calcitonin does not have a significant role in the homeostasis of plasma calcium in normal individuals. Other systemic effects of calcitonin include inhibition of insulin, growth hormone, prolactin, and gastrin secretion. When injected directly into the central nervous system, calcitonin depresses appetite and produces analgesia. Currently, nasal spray and injectable salmon calcitonin are approved in the United States as safe and effective for the treatment of hypercalcemia of malignancy, Paget's disease of bone, and late postmenopausal osteoporosis. Eel calcitonin has also been used effectively in this regard in Pacific-rim countries such as Japan, China, and Korea.

INJECTABLE CALCITONIN IN POSTMENOPAUSAL OSTEOPOROSIS

Salmon calcitonin was initially available as an injectable preparation. Initial data which led to approval of injectable calcitonin by the U.S. FDA in 1984 was the finding that injectable calcitonin given daily or every other day at 50 to 100 international units (IU) increased lumbar spine bone mass (BMD) by 2–3% in postmenopausal women with no associated deleterious effects on histologic properties of bone. However, the inconvenience of injection and side effects limited the widespread use of injectable calcitonin. The most common side effects of injectable calcitonin include nausea with or without vomiting, local reactions at the injection site, and flushing of the face and hands. These side effects are usually mild, dose dependent, and much more severe when calcitonin is given intramuscularly (i.m.) rather than subcutaneously, because of the higher blood calcitonin levels achieved during i.m. administration.

Early studies with injectable calcitonin in relatively poorly controlled studies demonstrated vertebral fracture reduction when 100 IU of the calcitonin plus 500 mg of calcium was administered for 10 days each month for 24 months. The latter was associated with a 12% increase in cortical bone mass and a 16% increase of spinal bone mass. In 1992, the results of a nonrandomized epidemiology European (MEDOS) study were also consistent with a greater tendency for injectable forms of salmon calcitonin to reduce hip fracture rates when compared to calcium alone. Observations demonstrating that patients with "high turnover" forms of osteoporotic bone disease who were rapidly losing bone respond dramatically well to calcitonin were consistent with its rapid effects on destroying osteoclastic activity in bone (Fig. 9-1).

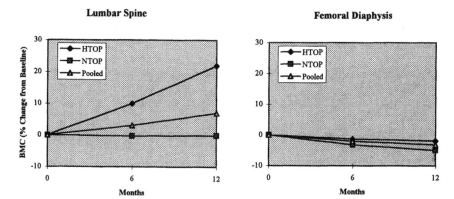

Fig. 9-1. Percent changes in BMC of the lumbar spine (left) and femoral diaphysis (right), in relation to bone turnover, in a group of postmenopausal women treated with salmon calcitonin for 1 year. BMC, bone mineral content; HTOP, high turnover osteoporosis; NTOP, normal turnover osteoporosis. (Adapted from The Journal of Clinical Investigation, 1988, 82, 1274, by copyright permission of The American Society for Clinical Investigation.)

NASAL SPRAY SALMON CALCITONIN

Calcitonin has been available as a nasal spray preparation in the United States since 1995. The nasal spray offers decreased side effects compared to the injectable formulation and has been generally well tolerated. The bioavailability of nasal calcitonin is not dose dependent and is about 25% of the administered dose as compared to the 70% bioavailability of the intramuscular preparation. An average dose of 200 IU of the nasal spray form of salmon calcitonin is equivalent to approximately 30–80 IU of the injectable preparation. A single dose of the calcitonin has rapid biological effects, resulting in transient hypocalcemia and occasionally phosphaturia, increased blood parathyroid hormone, increased urinary calcium, and increased circulating β-endorphins. Although the rise in plasma calcitonin following nasal spray administration is slower than observed with the injectable form, the plasma calcitonin level is sustained at a higher level for a longer period with the nasal spray formulation. Nasal spray calcitonin was approved in 1995 by the U.S. FDA and licensed by a variety of international agencies as safe and effective for the treatment of postmenopausal osteoporosis.

EFFICACY OF NASAL CALCITONIN IN POSTMENOPAUSAL OSTEOPOROSIS (EARLY STUDIES)

In 1989, Overgaard *et al.* randomized 40 late postmenopausal women with a history of prior forearm fractures to either 200 IU nasal spray calcitonin daily or placebo. All patients received 500 mg calcium daily. Valid completers who received a daily dose of 200 IU nasal spray calcitonin had a significant increase in lumbar spine BMD of 3.2% compared with the placebo group who lost (0.4%) bone. There was no significant difference between nasal spray calcitonin and placebo in both distal and proximal forearm BMD or total body bone mineral content among valid completers. In 1992, Overgaard *et al.* studied 208 females between the ages of 68 and 72 with low forearm bone density. Patients were randomized to placebo or 50, 100, or 200 IU calcitonin nasal spray daily for 2 years. All patients received 500 mg of calcium daily. Valid completers who received 200 IU nasal spray calcitonin demonstrated a significant increase in lumbar spine BMD of 3.0% in 24 months of study versus those treated with calcium only who had a mean increase of only 1%. In this study, 76% of patients treated with 200 IU of the nasal spray formulation responded to treatment, as defined by an increase in BMD when compared to baseline values, while only 38% of the placebo patients responded. Patients who received lower doses of nasal spray calcitonin did not show a significant increase in BMD. There was also a significant dose-related response to nasal spray calcitonin with an increase in lumbar spine BMD as compared to baseline of 1.0% for each 100 IU of calcitonin administered. Although this study was not designed to analyze the effect of therapy on fracture incidence, the rate of patients with new fractures was reduced significantly in valid completers in all groups taking nasal spray calcitonin to about one-third of the rate seen in the women who were only receiving calcium supplements. In subsequent studies, Ellerington (1996) compared two different regimens of 200 IU nasal spray calcitonin, daily versus intermittent (Monday, Wednesday, Friday) for 2 years in both early and late postmenopausal women. No calcium supplementation was given. There was no significant increase in lumbar spine BMD in patients who took calcitonin intermittently or in patients who took placebo although a significant increase in lumbar spine BMD in the late postmenopausal women was observed as early as 6 months in individuals on continuous therapy. At the end of 2 years in the more elderly postmenopausal patients receiving daily calcitonin doses of 200 IU, there was a significant increase in lumbar spine bone mass of 1.38% when compared to the untreated group who actually lost 1.73% of the baseline BMD (Table 9-1).

In 1997, a meta-analysis by Cardona and Pastor of published clinical trials designed to analyze the effects of calcitonin showed an "average" pooled change in vertebral BMD of 1.97% and a pooled change in femoral neck BMD of 0.32%. The aggregated number of vertebral fractures prevented by treatment was 59.2 per 1000 person years.

THE PROOF FIVE YEAR FRACTURE STUDY

The PROOF study (Prevent Recurrence of Osteoporotic Fractures) is as yet an unpublished multicenter double-blind randomized study of the effi-

TABLE 9-1. Changes in Lumbar Spine (DPA) BMD on Salmon Calcitonin Nasal Spray in Late Postmenopausal Women

Treatment group	Baseline mean BMD ± S.D.	Mean % change BMD			
		6 mo	12 mo	18 mo	24 mo
200 IU daily	1.10 ± 0.12 gm/cm^2	1.2%[a]	1.0%[a]	1.1%	1.4%[b]
200 IU MWF	1.09 ± 0.10	−0.4	−1.0	−0.5	−1.1
Placebo	1.11 ± 0.11	−1.2	−1.2	−1.1	−1.7[c]

Note: From Ellerington (1996).
[a]$P<0.025$ between group comparison.
[b]$P<0.01$ between group comparison.
[c]$P<0.01$ within group comparison.

cacy of salmon nasal spray calcitonin in the prevention of osteoporotic vertebral fractures. In the study, 1255 postmenopausal women, mean age 68, with established osteoporosis as defined by prior vertebral compression fracture or spine BMD at least 2 S.D. below normal for young premenopausal women were recruited in both the United States and United Kingdom. Women were randomized to placebo, 100, 200, or 400 IU of nasal spray daily, and all received supplements of 1000 mg elemental calcium and 400 IU of vitamin D per day. Using an intent to treat analysis and all accrued data through year 5 in the women with prevalent fracture, significant vertebral fracture reduction was demonstrated in women treated with 200 IU daily with a relative risk of new vertebral fracture compared to placebo of 0.64, representing a 36% fracture reduction (Chesnut 1998a). There was a 45% decrease in the number of women with multiple fractures and a 45% decrease in the rate of new vertebral fractures per 1000 person years in the 200 IU calcitonin treated group. The number of patients with two or more vertebral fractures was also 35% lower in individuals treated with 200 IU when compared to placebo. In these patients a mean decrease in the urine N-teleopeptide marker of bone resorption of 15–20% was observed at 12 months (Chesnut 1998a). The PROOF study was not powered to detect nonvertebral fracture reduction, although a 51% reduction in hip/femur fractures and 28% reduction in humerus/wrist fractures were observed, neither of which reached significance when compared to the untreated individuals (Chesnut 1998a).

Results of the PROOF study demonstrate that 200 IU nasal spray salmon calcitonin safely reduces the risk of new vertebral compression fractures over 5 years in postmenopausal women with established osteoporosis. Reduction in vertebral fracture risk was independent of baseline variables previously noted to influence fracture risk and response to calcitonin such as age, years since menopause, number of prevalent fractures, bone markers, and spinal BMD (Chesnut 1998b).

MECHANISM OF EFFECT OF CALCITONIN ON VERTEBRAL FRACTURE REDUCTION

Nasal spray calcitonin reduces the risk of vertebral fracture as shown in the PROOF study but the mechanism is still unclear. As noted for other agents that decrease fracture rates such as the SERM drug raloxifene, the effect of calcitonin on bone mineral density is modest as is the effect on urinary markers of bone resorption after 1 year of therapy. The mechanism(s) of action of antiresorptive therapies in preventing fracture include a decrease in bone turnover, increase in bone mass, and improved bone mineralization. It is also possible that nasal spray salmon calcitonin achieves a threshold level of increased BMD and decreased bone resorption which is sufficient to decrease erosion depth and trabecular perforation or improves bone quality by mechanisms yet undefined. In this regard, Gonnelli *et al.* (1996) showed a significant increase in the calcaneal stiffness using ultrasound in a group of patients taking 200 IU nasal calcitonin daily for alternate months for 2 years (Fig. 9-2). Since ultrasound stiffness predicts fracture risk more closely than correlation to BMD alone, the effects of calcitonin may be dependent on improvements in bone quality as well as BMD.

Stiffness

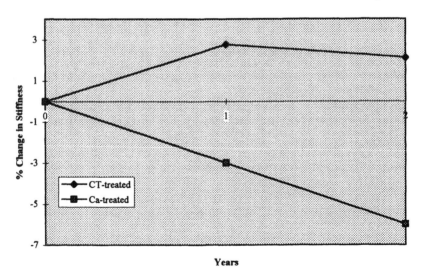

Fig. 9-2. Percent change in stiffness following 2 years of treatment with salmon calcitonin plus calcium, or calcium alone. Adapted with permission from Gonnelli, Cepollaro C, Pondrelli C, Martini S, Rossi S, Gennari C: Osteoporosis Int 6:303–307, 1996.

USE IN EARLY POSTMENOPAUSAL WOMEN TO PREVENT BONE LOSS

The efficacy of calcitonin in prevention of early postmenopausal bone loss has not been proven. A few studies have shown the possible efficacy of injectable calcitonin in the prevention of early postmenopausal bone loss at doses of at least 50 IU weekly. Limited studies have shown that 200–400 IU of nasal spray salmon calcitonin may slow down the rate of early postmenopausal bone loss. However, Campodarve *et al.* (1995) in a large multicenter study found that nasal calcitonin at doses up to 200 IU was not sufficient to inhibit bone resorption in the early postmenopausal period in a majority of women tested.

ANALGESIC EFFECTS OF CALCITONIN

The biological mechanism(s) that condition the analgesic response to calcitonin is not known but is thought most likely to involve β-endorphins, prostaglandins, the cholinergic or serontonineregic systems, and specific opioid receptors in the central nervous system. Although studies defining the analgesic effects of calcitonin preparations in osteoporosis have often been open label and not well controlled, there have been a few double-blind placebo controlled studies of osteoporotic subjects which demonstrate significant analgesic effects. Pun and Chan (1989) studied the analgesic effect of intranasal salmon calcitonin in the treatment of osteoporotic vertebral fractures. Patients with one to four vertebral fractures were treated with either nasal spray calcitonin at 200 IU per day or placebo. A significant decrease in bone pain graded by a visual analog score was observed after 7 days in patients receiving salmon calcitonin which persisted during the 28 day trial (Fig. 9-3). A statistically significant reduction in the consumption of analgesic

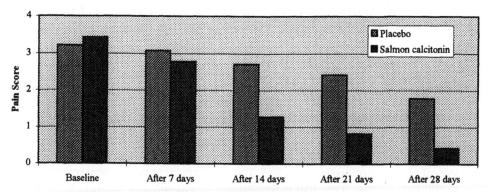

Fig. 9-3. Effect of intranasal salmon calcitonin and placebo on pain in patients with osteoporotic spinal fractures. Adapted by permission of the publisher from Pun KK, Chan LW: Clin Ther 11(2): 205–209. Copyright 1989 by Excerpta Medica Inc.

drugs was also observed as early as 7 days after treatment. Lyritis (1997) studied the analgesic effect of 200 IU nasal calcitonin in a double-blind placebo controlled study in patients with acute vertebral fracture(s) of less than 5 days duration using a visual analog scale for pain and patient assessment. Patients given calcitonin had significantly less back pain at rest, sitting, or standing by 1 week and significantly less back pain while walking at 2 weeks. There were also fewer bedridden patients in the calcitonin-treated group throughout the 4-week study. The accumulated data reveal that calcitonin is most effective for bone pain especially in patients with recent vertebral fractures.

ADMINISTRATION AND SIDE EFFECTS OF NASAL CALCITONIN

Nasal spray calcitonin is generally well tolerated. Common side effects include rhinitis, mild epistaxis, and headache. The incidence of gastrointestinal upset (<1.8%) and flushing (<1.0%) with nasal spray calcitonin are much lower than that observed with injectable calcitonin formulations. Because calcitonin is a protein, systemic allergic reactions are possible, although to date no allergic or anaphylactic reactions have been reported with the nasal spray formulation. There have been rare, isolated reports of anaphylaxis with injectable calcitonin and therefore skin testing is suggested in the product monograph. The author does not routinely skin test his patients before beginning treatment with nasal spray calcitonin.

The recommended dose of calcitonin nasal spray for the treatment of postmenopausal osteoporosis is 200 IU daily administered intranasally in alternating nostrils. The drug can be administered at any time, without regard to meals. In addition to calcitonin, patients should take adequate calcium (1000–1500 mg calcium) and 400 to 800 IU vitamin D every day. The medication should be refrigerated until opened, but then kept at room temperature and covered to avoid evaporation and condensation.

RESISTANCE TO CALCITONIN

Patients treated with calcitonin for long periods of time may develop clinical resistance. This has been observed in patients treated for Paget's disease in addition to patients with osteoporosis. As noted in the PROOF study, there was an approximate 1.2% increase in lumbar spine bone mass with a leveling off of the response in years 2–5. The mechanism of this clinical response is still not known. Two major hypotheses to explain calcitonin resistance have been production of antibodies and downregulation of osteoclast calcitonin receptor mRNA expression. Although an incidence of antibody formation of 50–65% to injectable calcitonin has been recorded, antibody titers may not necessarily accompanied by lack of drug efficacy. The fact that calcitonin resistance can also occur in the absence of antibodies confirms other reports that antibody formation to nasal spray calcitonin was not correlated with the skeletal response in patients with Paget's disease. A more likely explanation for clinical resistance to calcitonin may be the downregulation of hormonal receptors on osteoclasts following chronic exposure to the hormone. Takahashi *et al.* (1995) reported downregulation of calcitonin receptor mRNA expression by calcitonin during human osteoclast-like cell differentiation, a finding consistent with this hypothesis that intermittent exposure to calcitonin may avoid clinical resistance.

USE OF CALCITONIN IN COMBINATION THERAPY

Currently there is insufficient data regarding combination therapy using salmon calcitonin and any other drug in postmenopausal osteoporotic syndromes, although clinical efficacy with drug combinations may occur in patients with glucocorticoid-induced osteoporosis.

ROLE OF NASAL CALCITONIN IN THE THERAPY OF POSTMENOPAUSAL OSTEOPOROSIS

Nasal spray calcitonin should be considered as the initial treatment for the symptomatic osteoporotic patient with vertebral fractures and should be continued in those patients demonstrating clinical responses. Currently, nasal spray calcitonin formulations cannot be recommended for the prevention of osteoporosis in the early postmenopausal years. The drug is both safe and effective for patients with established osteoporosis not only in preventing recurrent vertebral fractures, but is also likely to be effective in controlling pain associated with morbid vertebral fracture syndromes.

SUMMARY AND CONCLUSIONS

Calcitonin is a safe treatment for established osteoporosis and has been available as an injectable preparation since 1984. Clinical trials over 28 years with either injectable or nasal spray forms of salmon calcitonin have demonstrated the efficacy of salmon calcitonin in increasing lumbar spine bone mass and decreasing vertebral fracture rates (nasal form) in patients with established osteoporosis. The use of injectable calcitonin has been limited by decreased compliance due to side effects and method of delivery. The availability (since 1995) of a nasal spray formulation with relatively few side effects as compared to placebo nasal spray has increased the convenience of use. Both injectable and nasal spray calcitonin demonstrate analgesic effects in osteoporotic individuals.

SUGGESTED READING

Azria M, Copp DH, Zanelli JM: Editorial: 25 years of salmon calcitonin: From synthesis to therapeutic use. Calcif Tissue Int 57:405–408, 1995.

Campodarve I, Drinkwater BL, Insogna KL, Johnston C, Lang R, Lindsay R, Neer R, Slovik DM, Gaich G, Procaccini R, Chesnut CH: Intranasal salmon calcitonin (INSC), 50–200 IU does not prevent bone loss in early postmenopausal women. J Bone Miner Res S391: C264, 1995 (abstract).

Cardona JM, Pastor E: Calcitonin versus etidronate for the treatment of postmenopausal osteoporosis: A meta-analysis of published clinical trials. Osteoporosis Int 7:165–174, 1997.

Chambers TJ, Moore A: The sensitivity of isolated osteoclasts to morphological transformation by calcitonin. J Clin Endocrinol Metab 57:819–824, 1983.

Chesnut C, Baylink DJ, Doyle D, Genant H, Harris S, Kiel DP, LeBoff M, Stock JL, Gimona A, Andriano K, Richardson P for the PROOF study group: Salmon calcitonin nasal spray prevents vertebral fractures in established osteoporosis. Further interim results of the Proof Study. Osteoporosis Int 8(Suppl 3):13, 1998a (abstract OR28).

Chesnut C, Silverman SL, Andriano K, Genant H, Richardson P, Maricic M, Stock J, Baylink D. Salmon calcitonin nasal spray reduces the rate of new vertebral fractures independently of known major pretreatment risk factors. Bone 23:5290, 1998b.

Civitelli R, Gonnelli S, Zacchei F, Bigazzi S, Vattimo A, Avioli LV, Gennari C: Bone turnover in postmenopausal osteoporosis: Effect of calcitonin treatment. J Clin Invest 82:1268–1274, 1988.

Cranney A, Moher D, Shea B, Wells G, Adachi R, Tugwell P: Metanalysis of calcitonin in the treatment of postmenopausal osteoporosis. Arth Rheum 38:S360–S369, 1995.

Deftos LJ: Medullary Thyroid Carcinoma. New York: Karger.

Ellerington MC, Whitcroft SIJ, Stevenson JC, Lees B, Marsh MS, Whitehead MI: Postmenopausal osteoporosis: A double-blind placebo-controlled study. Calcif Tissue Int 59:6–11.

Flicker L, Hopper JL, Larkins RG, Lichtenstein M, Vuirski G, Wark JD: Nandrolone decanoate and intranasal calcitonin as therapy in established osteoporosis. Osteoporosis Int 7:29–35, 1997.

Foti R, Martorana U, Broggini M: Long-term tolerability of nasal spray formulation of salmon calcitonin. Curr Ther Res 56:429–435, 1995.

Gennari C, Agnuddei D, Monatgnani M, Gonnelli S, Civitelli R: An effective regimen of intranasal salmon calcitonin in early postmenopausal bone loss. Calcif Tissue Int, 50:381–383, 1992.

Gonnelli S, Cepollaro C, Pondrelli C, Martini S, Rossi S, Gennari C: Ultrasound parameters in osteoporotic patients treated with salmon calcitonin: Longitudinal study. Osteoporosis Int 6:303–307, 1996.

Gruber HE, Ivey JL, Baylink DJ, Matthews M, Nelp WB, Sisom K, Chesnut CH III: Long-term calcitonin therapy in postmenopausal osteoporosis. Metabolism 33:295–303, 1984.

Healey JH, Paget SA, Williams-Russo P, Szatrowski TP, Schnedier R, Spiera H, Mitnick H, Ales K, Schwartzberg P: A randomized controlled trial of salmon calcitonin to prevent bone loss in corticosteroid-treated temporal arteritis and polymyalgia rheumatica. Calcif Tissue Int 58:73–80, 1996.

Hilton JM, Chai SY, Sexton PM: *In vitro* autoradiographic localization of the calcitonin receptor isoforms in rat brain. Neuroscience (Oxford) 69:1223–1237, 1995.

Kanis JA, Johnell O, Gulberg B, Allander E, Dilsen G, Gennari C, Lopez Vas AA, Lyritis BP, Mazzuoli G, Miravet L, Passeri M, Perez Cano R, Rapado A, Ribor C: Evidence for efficacy of drugs affecting bone metabolism in preventing hip fracture. Br Med J 305:1124–1128, 1992.

Kraenzlin ME, Seibel MJ, Trechsel U, Boerlin V, Azria M, Kraenzlin CA, Haas HG: The effect of intranasal salmon calcitonin on postmenopausal bone turnover as assessed by biochemical markers: Evidence of maximal effect after 8 weeks of continuous treatment. Calcif Tissue Int 58:216–220, 1996.

Lyritis GP, Paspati I, Karachalios T, Ioakimidis D, Skarantavos G, Lyritis PG: Pain relief from nasal salmon calcitonin in osteoporotic vertebral crush fractures. Acta Orthop Scand 68: (Suppl 275) 112–114, 1997.

MacIntyre I, Stevenson JC, Whitehead MI, Wimalawansa SJ, Banks LM, Healy MJR: Calcitonin for prevention of postmenopausal bone loss. Lancet 1:900–902, 1988.

Mannarini M, Fincato G, Galimberti S, Maderna M, Greco F: Analgesic effect of salmon calcitonin suppositories in patients with bone pain. Curr Ther Res 55:1079–1083, 1994.

Mazzuoli G, Passeri M, Gennari C, Minisola S, Atnonelli R, Valtrota C, Palummeri E, Cervellin S, Gonnelli S, Francini G: Effects of salmon calcitonin in postmenopausal osteoporosis: A controlled double-blind clinical study. Calcif Tissue Int 38:3–8, 1986.

Ongphiphadhanakal B, Piaseu N, Chailurkit L, Rajatanavin R: Suppression of bone resorption in early postmenopausal women by intranasal salmon calcitonin in relation to dosage and basal bone turnover. Calcif Tissue Int 62:379–382, 1998.

Overgaard K: Effect of intranasal salmon calcitonin therapy on bone mass and bone turnover in early postmenopausal women: A dose–response study. Calcif Tissue Int 55:82–86, 1994.

Overgaard K, Hansen MA, Nielsen VA, Riis BJ, Christiansen C: Discontinuous calcitonin treatment of established osteoporosis—effects of withdrawal of treatment. Am J Med 89:1–6, 1990.

Overgaard K, Agnusdei D, Hansen MA, Maioli E, Christiansen C, Gennari C: Dose response bioactivity and bioavailability of salmon calcitonin in premenopausal and postmenopausal women. J Clin Endocrinol Metab 72:344–349, 1991.

Overgaard K, Hansen MA, Jensen SB, *et al:* Effect of salcatonin given intranasally on bone mass and fracture rates in established osteoporosis: A dose response study. Br Med J 305:556–561, 1992.

Pontiroli AE, Pajetta E, Scaglia L, Rubinacci A, Resmini G, Arrigoni M, Pozza G: Analgesic effect of intranasal and intramuscular salmon calcitonin in postmenopausal osteoporosis: A double-blind, double placebo study. Aging Clin Exp Res 6:459–463, 1994.

Pun KK, Chan LW: Analgesic effect of intranasal salmon calcitonin in the treatment of osteoporotic vertebral fractures. Clin Ther 11:205–209, 1989.

Reginster JY, Gennari C, Mautalen C, Deroisy R, Denis D, Lecart MP, Vandalem JL, Collete J, Franchimont P: Influence of specific anti-salmon calcitonin antibodies on biological effectiveness of nasal salmon calcitonin in Paget's disease of bone. Scand J Rheum 19:83–86, 1990.

Resch H, Pietschmann P, Willvonseder R: Estimated long-term effect of calcitonin treatment in acute osteoporotic spine fractures. Calcif Tissue Int 45:209–213, 1989.

Rico H, Revilla M, Hernandez ER, Villa LF, Alvarez de Buergo M: Total and regional bone mineral content and fracture rate in postmenopausal osteoporosis treated with salmon calcitonin: A prospective study. Calcif Tissue Int 56:181–185, 1995.

Selander KS, Harkonen PL, Valve E, Monkkonen J, Hannuniemi R, Vaananen HK: Calcitonin promotes osteoclast survival *in vitro*. Mol Cell Endocrinol 122:119–129, 1996.

Silverman S, Chesnut C, Andriano K, Genant H, Gimona A, Maricic M, Stock J, Baylink D, for the PROOF study group: Salmon calcitonin nasal spray reduces risk of vertebral fracture in established osteoporosis and has a continuous effect with prolonged treatment: Accrued 5 year data of the PROOF Study. San Francisco: Presented at ASBMR, December 3, 1998.

Singer F, Alfred JP, Neer AM, Krane SM, Potts JT, Bloch KJ: An evaluation of antibodies and clinical resistance to salmon calcitonin. J Clin Invest 51:2331–2338, 1972.

Takahashi S, Goldring S, Katz M, Hilsenbeck S, Williams R, Roodman GD: Down-regulation of calcitonin receptor mRNA expression by calcitonin during human osteoclast-like cell differentiation. J Clin Invest 95:167–171, 1995.

Thamsborg G, Jensen JEB, Kollerup G, Hauge EM, Melsen F, Sorensen OH: Effect of nasal salmon calcitonin on bone remodeling and bone mass in postmenopausal osteoporosis. Bone 18:207–212, 1996.

Wallach S, Farley JR, Baylink DJ, Brenner-Gati L: Effects of calcitonin on bone quality and osteoblastic function. Calcif Tissue Int 52:335–3339, 1993.

Wimalawansa SJ: Long- and short-term side effects and safety of calcitonin in man: A prospective study. Calcif Tissue Int 52:90–93, 1993.

10 Therapy with Vitamin D Metabolites, Sodium Fluoride, Thiazides, and Isoflavones

Louis V. Avioli

VITAMIN D METABOLITES

The requirement that vitamin D must be biologically activated by the liver and kidney was initially demonstrated in experimental animals in 1967 and confirmed in humans in 1968. Subsequently, the primary biologically active metabolite, $1,25\text{-}(OH)_2D_3$ (calcitriol) was approved by the U.S. FDA for managing hypocalcemia and the associated metabolic bone disease in patients who are undergoing chronic renal dialysis, and for managing hypocalcemia in patients who have postsurgical hypoparathyroidism, idiopathic hypoparathyroidism, or pseudohypoparathyroidism. Calcitriol has not been approved in the United States specifically for treating osteoporosis although currently physicians prescribe it as "off label" use. A structurally related analogue $1\alpha\text{-}(OH)D_3$ (alfacalcidol) has also become available for this purpose outside the United States. The development of sensitive and precise blood assays for $25\text{-}(OH)D$ made it apparent that some postmenopausal and elderly osteoporotic females are prone to defective calcium absorption because of vitamin D deficiency (Table 10-1). The latter could result either from inadequate diets, poor sunlight exposure, and/or a decreased capacity of the skin of aging people to produce vitamin D_3. It was therefore considered appropriate by some to analyze the effects of treatment regimens using either $1,25\text{-}(OH)_2D_3$ or $1\text{-}(OH)D_3$ on the progression of the bone loss and the incidence of fractures in postmenopausal females. Observations made on patients receiving these agents range from those demonstrating ability to either increase bone mass and decrease vertebral (Fig. 10-1) and hip fracture incidence, to

**TABLE 10-1. Effect of Vitamin D and Calcium Therapy
on Bone Turnover in D-Deficient Elderly Women**

Variable[a]	Baseline	After 6 Months of Treatment
25-(OH)D (ng/ml)	3.0 ± 0.3	14.4 ± 0.1*
iPTH	39.0 ± 4.0	25.8 ± 3.0*
AP (IU)	84.8 ± 6.5	78.1 ± 8.7**
BAP (ng/ml)	12.5 ± 2.0	9.3 ± 1.3*
Hyp/Cr (µmol/mmol)	33.5 ± 8.4	23.4 ± 5.0**

Adapted from J Bone Miner Res 1995; 10:1753–1761, with permission of the American Society for Bone and Mineral Research.
[a]iPTH, circulating parathyroid hormone; BAP, circulating bone alkaline phosphatase as a biomarker for increased bone turnover; Hyp/Cr, urinary hydroxyproline as a biomarker for bone resorption. $*p < .0001.$ $**p < .01.$

reports of no change in bone mass and increased incidence of vertebral fracture, sustained hypercalciuria, and increases in serum calcium levels. Proponents of 1,25-$(OH)_2D_3$ [or 1α-$(OH)D_3$] treatment for osteoporotic fracture prone individuals argue that elevations in serum and urinary calcium result

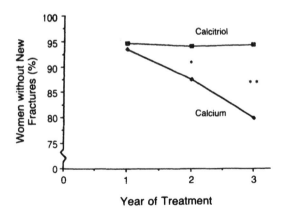

Fig. 10-1. Proportion of women treated with calcitriol, 1,25-$(OH)_2D_3$, or calcium who did not have a new vertebral fracture during a 3-year treatment period using 0.25 µg of calcitriol daily. The calcium-treated group received 1 g of Ca in the form of 5.2 g of calcium gluconate twice a day. The single asterisk (*) denotes significance of $p < .01$ after 2 years of treatment, a double asterisk (**) denotes significance of $p < .001$ after 3 years of treatment. In this study, the 24-h urinary calcium excretion was also significantly higher ($p < .001$) in the calcitriol-treated group (mean of 5.7 mmol/day) when compared to the calcium-treated group (mean 4.1 mmol/day). (Adapted from N Engl J Med 326:357, 1992. Copyright © 1992 Massachusetts Medical Society. All rights reserved.)

primarily from the use of large doses of these agents (i.e., 0.75–1.0 μg/day), and the failure to monitor and limit calcium intake. With 1,25-$(OH)_2D_3$ daily doses of 0.25 μg in osteoporotic females on controlled calcium intakes of 500–550 mg/day, hypercalciuria and hypercalcemia can apparently be minimized. In fact, cummulated data on 13,550 osteoporotic Oriental women who received 1α-$(OH)D_3$ for a minimum of 6 years demonstrated that the total frequency of side effects was 1.1% and that only 0.2% of subjects developed hypercalcemia. Thus, titration of the agent at the start of treatment is obligitory in order to obtain the optimum individual doses. Moreover, if these drugs are used to treat osteoporotic populations, there is a need to carefully monitor dietary calcium, especially in nonoriental populations who routinely consume diets containing 2–3 times the amount of calcium found in oriental foods. It should also be appreciated that subtle and progressive precipitation of calcium which can occur in cardiac and renal tissue of elderly patients with intermittent hypercalcemia and/or chronic hypercalciuria may contribute to cardiac arrhythmias and nephrocalcinosis. Consequently, if the chronic use of calcitriol or alfacalcidol is assumed, physicians must recognize that the window between achieving therapeutic benefits with the drug and hypercalciuria is small and that the side effects are most probably dose-dependent especially in patients who are not calcium restricted.

SODIUM FLUORIDE

It has been well-established that the fluoridation of municipal water supplies with as little as one part per million (ppm) of fluoride (1.0 mg/liter) results in an increased resistance to dental caries if the water is ingested during the first 12–13 years of life when the dentine and enamel of the permanent dentition are formed. There is also evidence that there are fewer vertebral fractures in endemic U.S. populations ingesting potable water during their lifetime containing fluoride in doses of 4–5 ppm, when compared to adjacent endemic areas with much less fluoride in the water supply (Fig. 10-2). The normal human skeleton does accumulate fluoride with age, and the fluoride concentration tends to be higher in males than in females of comparable ages. For many years there has been much optimism for the use of fluoride therapy in vertebral crush fracture syndromes based not only on these latter observations but also on reports of increased skeletal mass in individuals with the fluoride-intoxication syndrome known as "fluorosis," in malignant syndromes subjected to fluoride therapy, and a panoply of uncontrolled observations leading to testimonials of reductions either in vertebral fracture rates or vertebral "deformities" in fluoride-treated osteoporotic subjects. In fact, the ever increasing volume of data from at least five randomized control trials demonstrate increments in vertebral bone density in 70–75% of subjects receiving fluoride drugs, and histological increments in new

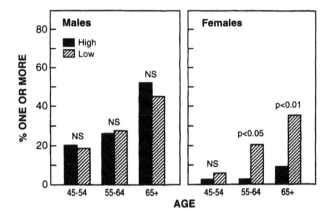

Fig. 10-2. Percentage of one or more collapsed vertebrae in subjects from high- and low-fluoride areas. (Adapted from JAMA 198 No. 5, Oct 31, 1966. Copyright 1966, American Medical Association.)

bone formation. Reports of low-dose slow release sodium fluoride related decreases in vertebral fracture incidence by 50%, resulted in approval of fluoride therapy for osteoporosis in some countries. At the time of this writing fluoride treatment that is not approved in the United States for the treatment of osteoporosis was approved by at least eight international communities (i.e., Austria, Belgium, France, Germany, Luxenbourg, The Netherlands, Norway, and Switzerland), despite continued lack of concurrence regarding efficacy and safety of chronic fluoride therapy.

There is currently general agreement that the majority of adult patients with osteoporotic syndromes will respond to fluoride administrations with an increment in vertebral bone mass, although for unknown reasons it is also not possible to predict which patient will respond in this manner. There is also a general consensus that side effects of fluoride therapy can be rather severe with gastrointestinal (nausea, vomiting, and gastrointestinal bleeding, with anemia) and/or lower extremity pain with arthralgias and "fatigue" fractures, and osteomalacia occurring in 10–40% of patients treated with this agent. Because appendicular (i.e., cortical) bone content can decrease during sodium fluoride therapy, and isolated reports of increased hip fracture frequency in individuals taking fluoride, enthusiasm has lessened for this agent as "therapeutic" in elderly populations. Although the unwanted effects observed during fluoride treatment are dose related and much more common with simple sodium fluoride preparations than with either enteric coated tablets, slow-release preparations, or intestinal-release preparations such as sodium monofluorophosphate, the long-term safety of flouride is still an issue and precludes the routine acceptance of this form of treatment for osteoporotic disorders until more definitive data become available.

THIAZIDE DIURETICS

Since thiazide therapy insures the retention of urinary calcium, these diuretics have been advocated as relatively safe and effective means of minimizing calcium loss, and presumably decreasing bone loss in the process (Fig. 10-3). Retrospective analyses of fracture profiles of elderly hypertensive populations on thiazide therapy for 6 or more years reveal a 30% decrease in hip fracture incidence, with the fracture risk decreasing significantly with increased duration of thiazide usage. More recently, the results of a 3-year randomized double-blind controlled study in 115 men and 205 women ages 60–79 years, revealed that hydrochlorothiazide in doses of 12.5 or 25 mg/day prevented bone loss.

The direct effects of thiazide diuretic drugs on bone are still ill-defined. However, since this family of diuretics can inhibit the activity of carbonic anhydrase (in the kidney) it is remotely possible that bone resorption is also

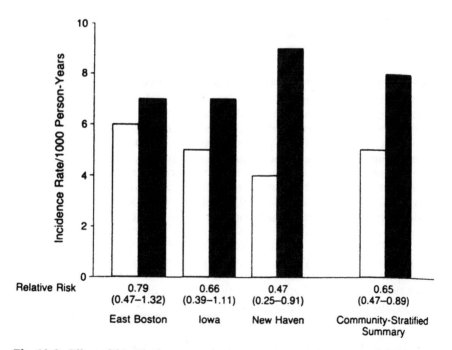

Fig. 10-3. Effect of thiazide therapy on fracture incidence. Rates are based on data obtained from 9518 subjects from three communities followed for up to 4 years. White bars represent thiazide users and dark bars, nonusers. Values in parentheses are 95% confidence intervals. (Reproduced from La Croix Az *et al:* N Engl J Med 322:286–290, 1990. Copyright © 1990 Massachusetts Medical Society. All rights reserved.)

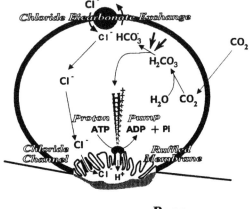

Bone

Fig. 10-4. Cartoon detailing the role of the osteoclast carbonic anhydrase (double arrows) as an enzyme that is pivotal in generating hydrogen ions (H^+) and bicarbonate ($HCO_3 -$) from H_2CO_3. When released together with chloride (Cl^-) ions from the osteoclast ruffled membrane, the H^+ (by a proton pump) produces the acidic environment essential for bone resorption.

inhibited. In this regard, we should be reminded that the skeletal osteoclastic resorption phenomenon is dependent on the production of hydrogen ions from carbon dioxide and water within the osteoclast. These hydrogen ions are then extruded from the cell, acidify the immediate extracellular domains of the osteoclast, and in the process "dissolve" the bone in the immediate vicinity (Fig. 10-4). The carbonic anhydrase enzyme, which generates hydrogen ions in the renal tubule from the carbon dioxide and water, functions in an identical fashion in the osteoclast. For this reason specific inhibitors of carbonic anhydrase activity, developed years ago and initially used as diuretics (i.e., Diamox), have proven to be very effective inhibitors of bone resorption in both *in vivo* experimental models of osteoporosis and in humans. Thiazides may also decrease the role of bone loss by directly stimulating osteoblast activity, and indirectly by suppressing calcium loss.

Despite these observations, with a drug that is cheap and often used as a first order defense in hypertensive populations, physicians should be cautious at this time in advocating thiazide therapy for nonhypertensive osteoporotic populations on a routine basis. The overall risk/benefit ratio of prolonged ingestion of thiazide diuretics must be considered, particularly with reference to hypercholesterolemic, hyperuricemic, hypercalcemic, and hypokalemic syndromes, as well as reported increments in urinary magnesium excretion and central nervous system symptoms which, not infrequently, accompany these metabolic derangements. Clinical awareness of these potential alterations in metabolic and mineral homeostasis is imperative especially with respect to magnesium, since the severity of magnesium depletion produced by thiazide-type diuretics rarely presents the classic magnesium deficiency syndrome with tetany and neuromuscular irritability. Moreover, although low levels of serum magnesium are almost always associated with tissue and/or whole body depletion of this element, tissue depletion of magnesium may occur during chronic thiazide-diuretic therapy despite normal blood levels. Diuretic-induced depletion of body magnesium is becoming of increasing concern to clinicians because of the relationship of hypomagnesemia, refractory potassium depletion, ventricular ectopy, and cardiac arrhythmias. When cardiac arrhythmias are observed in elderly patients on potassium-losing diuretics despite normal blood potassium levels, physicians should be aware of the possibility of a combined deficiency of magnesium and potassium. This association is especially noteworthy in the elderly who are predisposed to cardiac problems and who, either because of decreased intakes of magnesium due to decreased appetite, or the selection of foods with low magnesium content, are prone to chronic subclinical magnesium-deficient states.

ISOFLAVONES AND PHYTOESTROGENS

Many regimens recommended as "therapeutic" for osteoporotic individuals are still ignored by physicians. They either have restricted dosage schedules, unwanted clinical side effects, undesirable alteration in bone remodeling, and/or limited administration to early postmenopausal females. The ideal drug for either preventing or treating osteoporosis should be administered with minimal restrictions, be well-tolerated, prove therapeutic for both young postmenopausal women with "high-turnover" osteoporosis destined to lose bone rapidly and older women with established osteoporosis, and have little if any medical contraindications to routine use. Ideally, the drug of choice should also not accumulate in the skeleton where it could ultimately prove detrimental to normal bone turnover.

In this regard ipriflavone (7-isopropoxy-isoflavone) has been advocated by some as an alternative and favorable approach for either preventing or treating osteoporosis. Ipriflavone is an isoflavone-derived molecule that, like estrogens, functions primarily to suppress bone resorption although stimulation of bone cell growth and differentiation have also been documented during *in vitro* studies. Not only has ipriflavone proved beneficial in inhibiting bone turnover in patients with hyperparathyroidism and Paget's disease of bone, but therapeutic effects have been observed in either the axial and appendicular skeleton of oophorectomized women or others with ovarian suppression induced by GHRH agents. Ipriflavone in doses of 400–600 mg per day has been shown to prevent bone loss in young postmenopausal women as well as in more elderly osteoporotic individuals with low bone mineral density and established fracture syndromes.

To date, these results have been associated with a relatively favorable risk/benefit ratio and no significant difference in the frequency of adverse reactions when compared with placebo-treated control subjects. Moreover, although ipriflavone does share structural similarities with natural-occurring phytoestrogens, it does not exert estrogenic effects in the hypothalamus and pituitary gland. Ipriflavone not only increases bone mineral density when used alone but the drug is also effective in preventing early postmenopausal bone loss in patients treated with low doses of estrogens which, although ineffective in retarding bone loss, are sufficient to reduce the incidence of hot flushes and other characteristic postmenopausal symptoms. Although one can reasonably assume that the repeatedly observed effects of ipriflavone in stopping or decreasing the rate of axial and appendicular bone loss represent therapeutic efficacy that would ultimately lead to a significant decrease in the risk of osteoporotic fractures, we await the results of a multicenter, European, placebo-controlled, ipriflavone-fracture study in 460 postmenopausal women with established osteoporosis before this assumption can be considered an appropriate conclusion.

Phytoestrogens, which are plant compounds with estrogen like biological activity, have been considered by some as appropriate agents for preventing bone loss in women who cannot or will not comply to long-term estrogen regimens. Although a variety of foods contain phytoestrogens (Table 10-2), most clinical trials have been performed with soy-containing foods that contain the isoflavones, genestein and daidzein which are less than 1% as potent as circulating estrogens in binding assays (Table 10-2). However, despite the weak binding of these phytoestrogens to receptors

TABLE 10-2. Phytoestrogen Content Calculated from Results of Several Analyses

Food	Number of Foods Analyzed	Isoflavones	
		Daidzein (μg/g wet wt.)	Genestein (μg/g wet wt.)
Tofu	15	76	166
Soy sauce	3	8	5
Soy milk	10	18	26
Soy-based speciality formula	3	<1	3
Soybean sprouts	3	138	230
Soybean, green	1	546	729
Tempeh	3	190	320
Soybean paste	6	159	171
Miso paste	2	266	376
Miso paste (rice or barley)	3	79	260
Soy hot dog, tempeh burger	2	49	139

Adapted from Reinli K, Block G: Nutr Cancer 26:123–148, 1996. Copyright © 1996 Lawrence Erlbaum Associates, Inc.

TABLE 10-3. Effects of Phytoestrogens on Menopausal Hot Flashes

Investigator (year)	Phytoestrogen	Number of Patients	Statistics[a]
Murkies (1995)	45 g soy flour	58	↓ $p < .001$
Dalais (1996)	45 g linseed	52	↓ $p < .02$
Harding (1996)	80 mg soy protein (drink)	20	↓ $p < .03$
Brezezinski (1996)	80 g tofu miso 10 g linseed	165	↓ $p < .004$
Dalais (1996)	45 g soy grit enriched bread	52	NS

[a]A downward pointing arrow (↓) indicates a decreased incidence of hot flashes; NS, not significant.

that are essential for biological responses to estrogens, these dietary agents often produce a biological response comparable to those observed in women on estrogen therapy. In this regard, significant improvements in the vaginal maturation index and the incidence of hot flashes (Table 10-3) have been observed in women on diets containing 45 g of soy flour or 60 g of soy protein per day respectively.

Soy protein (i.e., genistein) isolates are equivalent to estrogens in preserving bone density in rodent models of osteoporosis, although the biological response may result from mechanisms which do not reflect estrogen activity on bone: that is, whereas estrogens suppress osteoclasts induced bone resorption, genistein appears to stimulate bone growth. Although studies in humans are relatively sparse, a recent 6-month randomized study using diets with high soy protein content (equivalent to 56–90 mg isoflavones per day) in postmenopausal women aged 49–73 years, revealed a 2% gain in vertebral bone mineral content when compared to a control group on milk protein diet. Similar results have not been obtained in women who were on diets containing calcium enriched soy milk (of unknown content) for 1 year, nor in ovariectomized monkeys, although beneficial effects of the soy enriched diets were observed on the coronary arteries of the monkeys. Currently, the data are far too meager to recommend dietary soy or isoflavone supplements for either the prevention or treatment of osteoporotic syndromes in postmenopausal women.

FUTURE HORIZONS

Since currently all accepted forms of therapy for osteoporosis utilize drugs that decrease bone turnover and osteoclast-induced bone resorption, there is a crying need for a form of anabolic treatment which is both safe and effective in preserving bone mass and preventing fractures. Currently, the pri-

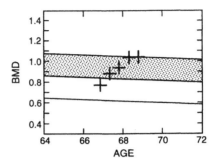

Fig. 10-5. Effect of daily PTH therapy on vertebral bone mineral density (BMD) in a 68-year-old female with osteoporosis. PTH therapy resulted in an 18% increase in BMD per annum in this individual. (Courtesy of C. Arnaud.)

mary candidate for this "anabolic agent" is parathyroid hormone (PTH). Studies in animals and humans reveal that in contrast to antiresorptive agents, PTH increases bone turnover with the latter resulting in significant increments in bone mineral density. Studies utilizing the 1–34 synthetic fragment of human PTH are currently ongoing in postmenopausal women and men with osteoporosis. With limited exceptions all demonstrate marked increments in vertebral bone mineral density (Fig. 10-5). In one study a reduction in the incidence of vertebral deformities has been recorded. Although additional clinical observations regarding safety, optimal dosing regimens, and extravertebral site responsivity to PTH are essential, delivery systems other than the prevailing current injection protocols including nasal sprays, pulmonary inhalation, and oral preparations are being pursued.

Since growth hormone (GH) deficiency appears to play a central role in the development of osteopenia in hypopituitary patients who have fracture frequencies approximately 2–3 times higher than appropriately matched populations, and because GH stimulates bone formation and longitudinal bone growth, this agent has also been tested as a potential anabolic agent for osteoporotic subjects. Results in GH-deficient individuals reveal a "biphasic" response to GH treatment with an initial 6-month bone resorption phase followed by a progressive increase in bone formation and bone mineralization with increments in bone mass determined by dual photon densitometry (DEXA) measurements observed after 12–18 months of therapy. Since this "biphasic" response has been noted in GH-deficient adults, the hormone cannot be currently recommended as "safe and effective" treatment for osteoporotic individuals with normal pituitary function. In fact when tested in a cyclical fashion in a small population of normal osteopenic women (i.e., lumbar spine bone mineral density <1 standard deviation (SD) below mean value for healthy 25-year-old women) for 2 years, mild increments in bone mass were attended by a panoply of adverse experiences that preclude the use of GH as a useful anabolic strategy in postmenopausal osteoporotic patients.

Finally, with respect to testosterone therapy in osteoporotic males, a recent study reveals that increasing serum testosterone concentrations of normal men over 65 years of age to the midnormal range for young men does not increase lumbar spine bone density, whereas testosterone administration did increase bone density in men with low pretreatment serum testosterone concentrations. Strong contraindications to testosterone therapy in females include enhanced libido, moderate to severe acne, hirsutism, and alopecia.

SUGGESTED READING

Vitamin D Metabolites

Aloia JF, Vaswani A, Yeh JK, Ellis KH, Yasumura S, Cohn SH: Calcitriol in the treatment of postmenopausal osteoporosis. Am J Med 84:491–498, 1988.

Bouillon RA, Auwerx JH, Lissens WD, Pelemans WK: Vitamin D status in the elderly: Seasonal substrate deficiency causes 1,25-dihydroxycholecalciferol deficiency. Am J Clin Nutr 45:755–763, 1987.

Jensen GF, Meinecke B, Boesen J, Transbol I: Does 1,25(OH)$_2$D$_3$ accelerate spinal bone loss? Clin Orthop 192:215–221, 1985.

Nishii Y, Sato K, Kobayashi T: The development of vitamin D$_3$ analogues for the treatment of osteoporosis. Osteoporosis Int 1:S190–S193, 1993.

Orimo H, Shiraki M, Hayashi T, Nakamura T: Reduced occurrence of vertebral crush fractures in senile osteoporosis treated with 1 (OH)-vitamin D$_3$. Bone Miner 3:47–52, 1987.

Ott SM, Chesnut CH III: Calcitriol treatment is not effective in postmenopausal osteoporosis. Ann Intern Med 110:267–274, 1989.

Tilyard MW, Spears GFS, Thompson J, Dovey S: Treatment of postmenopausal osteoporosis with calcitriol or calcium. N Engl J Med 326:357–361, 1992.

Utiger RD: Editorial: The need for more vitamin D. N Engl J Med 338:828–829, 1998.

Villareal DT, Civitelli R, Chines A, Avioli LV: Subclinical vitamin D efficiency in postmenopausal women with low vertebral bone mass. J Clin Endocrinol Metab 72:628–634, 1991.

Whyte MP, Haddad JG Jr, Walters DD, Stamp TCB: Variable potency of intracellular vitamin D preparations. N Engl J Med 300:142, 1979.

Sodium Fluoride

Dambacher MA, Ittner J, Ruegsegger P: Long-term fluoride therapy of postmenopausal osteoporosis. Bone 7:199–205, 1986.

De Deuxchaisnes CN, Devogelaer JP, Depresseux G, Malghem J, Maldague B: Treatment of the vertebral crush fracture syndrome with enteric-coated sodium fluoride tablets and calcium supplements. J Bone Miner Res 5:S5–S26, 1990.

Dure-Smith BA, Farley SM, Linkhart SC, Farley JR, Baylink DJ: Calcium deficiency in fluoride-treated osteoporotic patients despite calcium supplementation. J Clin Endocrinol Metab 81:269–275, 1996.

Kleerekoper M, Balena R: Fluorides and osteoporosis. Annu Rev Nutr 11:309–324, 1991.

Madans J, Kleinman JC, Cornoni-Huntley J: The relationship between hip fracture and water fluoridation: An analysis of national data. Am J Public Health 73:296–298, 1983.

Pak CYC, Sakhaee K, Zerwekh JE, Parcel C, Peterson R, Johnson K: Safe and effective treatment of osteoporosis with intermittent slow release sodium fluoride: Augmentation of vertebral bone mass and inhibition of fractures. J Clin Endocrinol Metab 68:150–159, 1989.

Pak CYC, Sakhaee K, Adams-Huet B, Piziak V, Peterson RD, Pointdexter JR: Treatment of postmenopausal osteoporosis with slow-release sodium fluoride. Ann Intern Med 123:401–408, 1995.

Reginster JY, Meurmans L, Zegels B, Rovati LC, Minne HW, Giacovelli G, Taquet A, Setnikar I, Collette J, Gosset C: The effect of sodium monofluorophosphate plus calcium on vertebral fracture rate in postmenopausal women with moderate osteoporosis. A randomized controlled trial. Ann Intern Med 129:1–8, 1998.

Riggs BL, Hodgson SF, O'Fallon M, Chao EYS, Wahner HW, Muhs JM, Cedel SL, Melton LJ III: Effect of fluoride treatment on the fracture rate in postmenopausal women with osteoporosis. N Engl J Med 322:802–809, 1990.

Riggs BL, O'Fallon WM, Lane A, Hodgson SF, Wahner HW, Muhs J, Chao E, Melton LJ III: Clinical trial of fluoride therapy in postmenopausal osteoporotic women: Extended observations and additional analysis. J Bone Miner Res 9:265–275, 1994.

Ringe JD, Kipshoven C, Coster A, Umbach R: Therapy of established postmenopausal osteoporosis with monofluorophosphate plus calcium: Dose-related effects on bone density and fracture rate. Osteoporosis Int 9:171–178, 1999.

Zerwekh JE, Padalino P, Pak CYC: The effect of intermittent slow-release sodium fluoride and continuous calcium citrate therapy on calcitropic hormones, biochemical markers of bone metabolism, and blood chemistry in postmenopausal osteoporosis. Calcif Tissue Int 61:272–278, 1997.

Thiazides

Adams JS, Song CF, Kantorovich V: Rapid recovery of bone mass in hypercalciuric, osteoporotic men treated with hydrochlorothiazide. Ann Intern Med 130:658–660, 1999.

Aubin R, Menard P, Lajeunesse D: Selective effect of thiazides on the human osteoblast-like cell MG-63. Kidney Int 50:1476–1482, 1996.

Cauley JA, Cummings SR, Seeley DG: Effects of thiazide diuretic therapy on bone mass fractures and falls. Ann Intern Med 118:666–673, 1993.

Chang SW, Fine R, Siegel D, Chesney M, Black D, Hulley SB: The impact of diuretic therapy on reported sexual function. Arch Intern Med 151:2402–2408, 1991.

Felson DT, Sloutskis D, Anderson JJ, Anthony JM, Kiel DP: Thiazide diuretics and the risk of hip fractures. Results from the Framingham study. JAMA 265:370–373, 1991.

Gluck S: The osteoclast as a unicellular proton-transporting epithelium. Am J Med Sci 303:134–139, 1992.

Heidrich FE, Stergachis A, Gross KM: Diuretic drug use and the risk for hip fracture. Ann Intern Med 115:1–6, 1991.

LaCroix AZ, Wienpahl J, White LR, Wallace RB, Scherr PA, George LK, Cornoni-Huntley J, Ostfeld AM: Thiazide diuretic agents and the incidence of hip fracture. N Engl J Med 322:286–290, 1990.

Martin BJ, Milligan K: Diuretic-associated hypomagnesemia in the elderly. Arch Intern Med 147:1768–1771, 1987.

Peh CA, Horowitz N, Wishart JM, Need AG, Morris HA, Nordin BEC: Effect of chlorothiazide on bone-related biochemical variables in normal and postmenopausal women. J Am Geratr Soc 41:513–516, 1993.

Pierce WM Jr, Nardin GF, Fuqua MF, Sabah-Maren E, Stern SH: Effect of chronic carbonic anhydrase inhibitor therapy on bone mineral density in white women. J Bone Miner Res 6:347–354, 1991.

Pollare T, Lithell H, Berne C: A comparison of the effects of hydrochlorthiazide and captopril on glucose and lipid metabolism in patients with hypertension. N Engl J Med 321:868–873, 1989.

Ray WA: Editorial: Thiazide diuretics and osteoporosis: Time for a clinical trial? Ann Intern Med 115:64–65, 1991.

Salem M, Kasinski N, Andrei AM, Brussel T, Gold MR, Conn A, Chernow B: Hypomagensemia is a frequent finding in the emergency department in patients with chest pain. Arch Intern Med 151:2185–2190, 1991.

Soers MR, Clark MK, Jannausch ML, Wallace RB: Body size, estrogen use and thiazide diuretic use affect 5-year radial bone loss in postmenopausal women. Osteoporosis Int 3:314–321, 1993.

Swales JD: Magnesium deficiency and diuretics. Br Med J 285:1377–1378, 1982.

Wasnich RD, Davis JW, He Y-F, Petrovich H, Ross PP: Randomized double-masked, placebo-controlled trial of chlorthalidone and bone loss in elderly women. Osteoporosis Int 5:247–251, 1995.

Whang R Whang DD, Ryan MP: Refractory potassium repletion. A consequence of magnesium deficiency. Arch Intern Med 152:40–45, 1992.

Isoflavones

Adami S, Bufalino L, Cervetti R, DiMarco C, DiMunno O, Fantasia L, Isaia C, Serni U, Vecchiet L, Passeri M: Ipriflavone prevents radial bone loss in postmenopausal women with low bone mass over 2 years. Osteoporosis Int 7:119–125, 1997.

Agnusdei D, Adami S, Cervetti R, Crepaldi G, DiMunno O, Fantasia L, Isaia GC, Letizia S, Ortolani S, Passeri M, Serni U, Vecchiet L, Gennari C: Effects of ipriflavone on bone mass and calcium metabolism in postmenopausal osteoporosis. Bone Miner 19:S43–S48, 1992.

Aoyagi K, Iwasaki K, Hayashi T, Inoue H, Yamaguchi K, Takahara K: Effect of ipriflavone in combination with calcium supplements on bone metabolism in elderly osteoporotic women. J Bone Miner Metab 14:79–82, 1996.

Arjmandi BH, et al: Dietary soybean protein prevents bone loss in an ovariectomized rat model of osteoporosis. J Nutr 126:161–167, 1996.

Avioli LV: The future of ipriflavone in the management of osteoporotic syndromes. Calcif Tissue Int 61:S33–S35, 1997.

Bufalino L, Abate G, Pedrazzoni M, Passeri M: Effect of 3-year treatment with ipriflavone on bone mass in women with severe osteoporosis. European Congress for Osteoporosis, Berlin, September 11–15, 1998 (abstract 255).

Civitelli R, Abbasi-Jarhomi H, Halstead LR, Dimaragonas A: Ipriflavone improves bone density and biomechanical properties of adult male rat bones. Calcif Tissue Int 56:215–219, 1995.

Clarkson TB, et al: The potential for soybean phytoestrogens for postmenopausal hormone replacement therapy. Proc Soc Exp Biol Med 217:365–368, 1998.

Fanti O, *et al*: Systematic administration of genistein partially prevents bone loss in ovariectomized rats in a nonestrogen-like mechanism. Am J Clin Nutr 68:1517, 1998 (abstract).

Gambacciani M, Spinetti A, Cappagli B, Taponeco F, Felipetto R, Parrini D, Cappelli N, Pioretti P: Effects of ipriflavone administration on bone mass and metabolism in ovariectomized women. J Endocrinol Invest 16:333–337, 1993.

Gambacciani M, Spinetti A, Piaggesi L, Cappagli B, Taponeco F, Manetti P, Weiss C, Teti GC, La Commare P, Facchini V: Ipriflavone prevents the bone mass reduction in premenopausal women treated with gonadotropin hormone-releasing hormone agonists. Bone Miner 26:19–26, 1994.

Honore EK, *et al*: Soy isoflavones enhance coronary vascular reactivity in atherosclerotic female macaques. Fertil Steril 67:148–154, 1997.

Lees CJ, Ginn TA: Soy protein isolate diet does not prevent increased cortical bone turnover in ovariectomized macaques. Calcif Tissue Int 62:557–558, 1998.

Maugeri D, Panebianco P, Russo MS, *et al*: Ipriflavone treatment of senile osteoporosis: Results of a multicenter, double-blind clinical trial of 2 years. Arch Gerontol Geriatr 19:253–263, 1994.

Melis GB, Paoletti AM, Cagnacci A, Bufalino L, Spinetti A, Gambacciani M, Fioretti P: Lack of any estrogenic effect of ipriflavone in postmenopausal women. J Endocrinol Invest 15:755–761, 1992.

Melis GB, Paoletti Am, Cagnacci A: Ipriflavone prevents bone loss in postmenopausal women. Menopause 3:27–32, 1996.

Murkies AL, Wilcox G, Davis SR: Phytoestrogens. J Clin Endocrinol Metab 83:297–303, 1998.

Olsen EL, *et al*: Bone gain after calcium enriched soy milk, food supplement, and lifestyle changes in women with low bone mass. A pilot project in course form. Am J Clin Nutr 68:1518, 1998 (abstract).

Passeri M, Biondi M, Costi D, *et al*: Effects of 2-year therapy with ipriflavone in elderly women with established osteoporosis. Ital J Miner Electrolyte Metab 9:137–144, 1995.

Potter SM, *et al*: Soy protein and isoflavones: Their effects on blood lipids and bone density in postmenopausal women. Am J Clin Nutr 68:1375–1379, 1998.

Valente M, Bufalino L, Castiglione GN, D'Angelo R, Mancuso A, Galoppi P, Zichella L: Effects of 1-year treatment with ipriflavone on bone in postmenopausal women with low bone mass. Calcif Tissue Int 54:377–380, 1994.

Future Horizons

Biller BMK: Efficacy of growth hormone-replacement therapy: Body comparison and bone density. The Endocrinologist 8:15S–21S, 1998.

Colao A, Di Somma C, Pivonello R, Loche S, Aimaretti G, Cerbone G, Faggiano A, Corneli G, Ghigo E, Lombardi G: Bone loss is correlated to the severity of growth hormone deficiency in adult patients with hypopituitarism. J Clin Endocrinol Metab 84:1919–1924, 1999.

Cosman F, Lindsay: Is parathyroid hormone a therapeutic option for osteoporosis? A review of the clinical evidence. Calcif Tissue Int 62:475–480, 1998.

Cosman F, Nieves J, Woelfert L, Gordon S, Shen V, Lindsay R: Parathyroid responsivity in postmenopausal women with osteoporosis during treatment with parathyroid hormone. J Clin Endocrinol Metab 83:788–790, 1998.

Davis S: Androgen replacement in women: A commentary. J Clin Endocrinol Metab 84:1886–1891, 1999.

Finkelstein JS, Klibanski A, Schaefer EH, Hornstein MD, Schiff I, Neer RM: Parathyroid hormone for the prevention of bone loss induced by estrogen deficiency. N Engl J Med 331:1618–1623, 1999.

Hirano T, Burr DB, Turner CH, Sata M, Cain RL, Hock JM: Anabolic effects of human biosynthetic parathyroid hormone fragment (1–34), LY333334, on remodeling and mechanical properties of cortical bone in rabbits. J Bone Miner Res 14:536–545, 1999.

Holloway L, Kohlmeier L, Kent K, Marcus R: Skeletal effects of cyclic recombinant human growth hormone and salmon calcitonin in osteopenic postmenopausal women. J Clin Endocrinol Metab 82:1111–1117, 1997.

Ohlsson C, Bengtsson BA, Isaksson OGP, Andreassen TT, Slootweg MC: Growth hormone and bone. Endocr Rev 19:55–79, 1998.

Rihani-Bisharat S, Maor G, Lewinson D: *In vivo* anabolic effects of parathyroid hormone (PTH) 28–48 and N-terminal fragments of PTH and PTH-related protein on neonatal mouse bones. Endocrinology 139:974–981, 1998.

Snyder PJ, Peachey H, Hannoush P, Berlin JA, Loh L, Holmes JH, Dlewati A, Staley J, Santanna J, Kapoor SC, Attie MF, Haddad JG, Strom BL: Effect of testosterone treatment on bone mineral density in men over 65 years of age. J Clin Endocrinol Metab 84:1966–1972, 1999.

11 Orthopedics and the Osteoporotic Syndrome

William J. Maloney

INTRODUCTION

Osteoporosis is a significant public health problem primarily because of its relationship to insufficiency fracture. As such, it impacts the practice of orthopedic surgery on a daily basis. Not only does this disease process affect the prevalence, pattern, and ability to surgically stabilize fractures; the orthopedic surgeon must also understand the impact that surgical intervention and disease processes may have on local bone metabolism. In this section, these issues will be reviewed.

OSTEOPOROSIS AND FRACTURE

Epidemiology

It has been estimated that osteoporosis affects approximately 25 million Americans. This is primarily a disease of the elderly and as the population of elderly continues to grow as a result of improved health care, it is likely that the prevalence of this disease will continue to increase. People over the age of 65 now constitute approximately 12.5% of the U.S. population.

The economic impact of this on health care is marked. It is estimated that 1.2 to 1.3 million fractures are annually attributed to osteoporosis. These include fractures of the vertebral column, hip, and distal radius as the most common sites. The risk of fracture increases with age. Women who live to the age of 90 have a 32% chance of developing a hip fracture. In men, the risk is 17%.

For the elderly patient that sustains a hip fracture, this represents a significant impact on their overall quality of life. Twelve to twenty percent of the elderly who sustain a hip fracture die within a year after fracture. Approximately half of these patients require long-term nursing care and only a small percentage are able to return to their prefracture ambulatory status. If a patient requires nursing home care following hip fracture, approximately 70% of those patients will die within 1 year.

From a financial standpoint, the magnitude of the problem is also marked. The elderly, including people over the age of 65, represent a significant percentage of patients currently occupying a hospital bed in this country. One in 20 of those patients who are older than 65 are hospitalized because of a hip fracture. Looking at hip fractures alone, the cost of treatment in the United States has been estimated at up to 10 billion dollars annually. From the standpoint of managing the health care budget, the importance of this becomes obvious.

Risk Factors

A variety of factors put patients at risk for osteoporosis, including age, hereditary factors, nutrition, and lifestyle, as well as medications. Bone loss with age is a normal phenomenon. Risk of fracture increases as bone mass decreases. The World Health Organization has defined osteoporosis as low bone density 2.5 standard deviations below the mean. From a functional standpoint, it is important that the relationship between osteoporosis and insufficiency fracture be clearly defined. As such, a person with two or more insufficiency fractures is considered to have severe osteoporosis. Based on these definitions, it is estimated that 30% of postmenopausal women have osteoporosis in the United States. The estrogen loss associated with menopause accelerates osteoporosis and is especially important in women who have early menopause or amenorrhea. From the standpoint of the orthopedic surgeon, one has to pay special attention to the young female athlete. Excessive exercise such as in long distance runners can often result in amenorrhea and can lead to severe osteoporosis. In addition, eating disorders such as anorexia nervosa can also induce amenorrhea and thus osteoporosis.

It is clear that hereditary factors also play a role. Small build, thin, fair-skinned women of Caucasian or Asian background have an increased risk for osteoporosis. Lifestyle in terms of nutrition and dietary intake of calcium as well as exercise or lack thereof have also been linked to osteoporosis. Smoking and excessive alcohol use are contributory. Medications can be important as a potential etiologic factor in the development of osteoporosis especially corticosteroids.

Pathophysiology of Fracture

There are two basic types of bone, cortical and trabecular. Trabecular bone is located primarily in the spinal column as well as in the metaphyseal region of the long bones. Trabecular bone is subjected primarily to impact type of stresses whereas a cortical bone sees torque and bending moments as its primary load.

In osteoporosis, trabecular bone tends to be lost first. As a result, those regions of the skeleton that are composed of a large amount of trabecular bone, are most commonly involved in pathologic fractures associated with osteoporosis. Thus, vertebral compression fractures are the most common fractures associated with osteoporosis. It is estimated that more than 500,000 vertebral fractures occur each year in the United States. One-third of all women over the age of 65 will have a vertebral compression type fracture. Vertebral fractures are followed by hip fracture and distal forearm, primarily distal radius fractures as the second and third most common related insufficiency type fracture.

Although there is obviously a relationship between bone density and fracture, bone density in and of itself is not the only important factor. The structure of bone as well as the tendency for a patient to fall and the ability of that patient to heal microfractures also play a role. There is, however, a correlation between fracture and bone mass. For vertebral fractures, it has been demonstrated that patients who develop compression fractures have significantly lower bone mass as measured by a dual beam absorptiometry. As the spinal bone mass decreases, fracture rate increases. For example, 86% of patients with a spinal bone mass of 0.8 and 0.9 g/cm^2 developed a fracture of the vertebral column. When bone mass decreased to 0.5 to 0.6 g/cm^2, the percentage of spinal fractures increased to 63%. However, this work also demonstrated that because of the overlap that existed between patients with and without a compression fracture of the spine, there was not a clear cutoff in terms of absolute risk for patients for developing this type of fracture. There are data which demonstrate that with a 50% decrease in bone mass, there is a 4-fold increase in the rate of developing a hip fracture.

Hip fracture is the most common insufficiency type fracture requiring surgical intervention. Approximately 90% of hip fractures in the elderly are associated with a fall. This fact alone points to the importance of looking at fall mechanics in the elderly as well as emphasizing programs to reduce the risk of fall in this patient population. Although fall is by far and away the most common etiologic factor in hip fracture in the elderly patient population, it is also important to remember that only about 2% of falls in the elderly result in hip fracture. Therefore, it is important not only to reduce the prevalence of falls, but also to identify the high-risk fall. To this end, investigators have categorized falls and defined fall as a sudden unexpected event that results in the person coming to rest on a horizontal surface. Falls have been divided into several states or phases including an instability phase resulting in fall initiation, a descent phase, and an impact phase, as well as a postimpact phase. In terms of risk for hip fracture, previous authors have defined a high-risk fall as a fall that results in impact on or near the hip, a fall in which there is a lack of an active protective mechanism, such as an outstretched arm, and a fall in which there is insufficient energy of absorption by local soft tissues to protect the hip joint. The result is a high impact load directly to the proximal femur resulting in a fracture of the hip.

This concept has been confirmed to some degree by surveillance studies which have tried to characterize falls and look at specific fall mechanics as they relate to whether or not a given individual develops a hip fracture. Women who suffer a hip fracture from a fall are more likely to have fallen sideways or straightforward landing on or near the hip. In addition women who have broken their hip with such a fall tended to be taller, had weaker upper extremity musculature, specifically tricep muscles, and were less likely to have broken the fall with an outstretched arm.

In terms of the biomechanics and vertebral fractures, this phenomenon has been less well investigated. As noted above, there is a correlation between bone mineral density and vertebral fracture. The role of spinal loading and degree to which the spine must be loaded to cause a fracture has not been studied extensively. Retrospective analyses in a patient population from Rochester, Minnesota, demonstrated that a specific event with loading of the spinal column was reported in only about 50% of the fractures. Interestingly, few of the fractures were related to lifting (10%). Thirty-nine percent of symptomatic vertebral compression fractures were reported as being spontaneous with no causative event. Thirty percent were associated with a fall from a standing height or less and an additional 9% were associated with a fall from a height of greater than standing height. Ten percent of vertebral compression fractures occurred from lifting heavy objects, 7% as a result of a traffic accident, and only 4% were pathologic fractures related to spinal neoplasms.

Biomechanical models have been developed to estimate the load on the spine during activities of daily living. Using these models, it has been estimated that simple activity such as rising from a chair can result in compressive forces on the spinal column from 60 to 173% of body weight depending on the level analyzed.

These models have also demonstrated the importance of body position on spinal load. For a given individual standing erect and holding an 8 kilogram weight with the arms slightly extended the compressive force on L2 was calculated to be approximately 230% of body weight. If the individual then flexed the trunk forward at an angle of 30° the compressive force on L2 increased to over 320% of body weight.

Based on the above discussion, the importance of falls as an etiologic factor in osteoporotic fractures is evident. As noted above, falls from a standing height or less are the most common mechanism of injury for hip fractures in the elderly patient population. Approximately half of these falls resulting in hip fracture are mechanical falls, that is, tripping or slipping. Other causes of falls include syncope, orthostatic hypotension, or simple loss of balance.

Loss of balance represents a compromise of the ability of the patient to maintain postural mechanics. Although balance and coordination may be modified by exercise programs in order to decrease falls, inadequate selection of appropriate programs and/or poor compliance by elderly populations often minimize the beneficial effects of the program. To maintain postural mechanics, there is a requirement for input from the visual system, vestibular system, as well as proprioceptors. With increasing age, all three decrease in terms of their function.

Three-quarters of femoral neck fractures occur indoors and environmental hazards contribute to two-thirds of these. Factors described above can be divided into intrinsic and extrinsic factors as they relate to falls. Intrinsic factors would include things like syncope, hypotension, drop attacks, and neurovascular incidents such as TIAs and strokes. Extrinsic factors are related to mechanical factors such as stairs, throw rugs, carpet edges, waxed floors, telephone cords, as well as inadequate lighting, particularly from well-traveled areas such as from the bedroom to the bathroom. The vast majority of elderly patients have nocturia which results in them getting out of bed two or more times per night to void. At this point, they are particularly vulnerable as they are awakening from sleep, they often have even poorer balance than when wide awake, and lighting is often a problem. Although hip padded protection devices have been used to prevent fractures in institutional patients (Table 11-1), the value of this preventative mode in free-standing mobile subjects still requires additional documentation.

Intrinsic factors can be increased by the use of medications. Particularly medications that are problematic in this regard include barbiturates, phenothiazine, antidepressants, long half-life benzodiazepines, and antihypertensives, including diuretics. In a recent review of changing incidences of hip

TABLE 11-1. External Hip Protectors and Hip Fractures

	Hip Protector Group ($n = 247$)	Controls ($n = 418$)	RR (95% CI)
Hip fractures	8	31	0.44 (0.01–0.94)[a]
Nonhip fractures	15[b]	27	0.94 (0.51–1.7)

Adapted from Lauritzen *et al:* Lancet 341:11, 1993. © by The Lancet Ltd.
[a]Age-adjusted RR = 0.41 (0.18–0.82).
[b]Fractures to upper limb; none to lower limb.

fracture in Sweden, a decrease in hip fracture incidence was associated with a decrease in the use of sedatives with "hangover effects."

Surgical Interventions

The most common indication for surgery in the face of osteoporosis is acute fragility or insufficiency of fracture requiring open reduction and internal fixation. Other relatively common surgical procedures required in the face of osteoporosis include total joint replacement and spinal stabilization. Osteoporosis is somewhat unique in that unlike osteomalacia or Paget's disease, medical management of osteoporosis does not enhance the healing potential of bone.

Fracture Management

There is a general opinion that "timing" is critical in the surgical and rehabilitative care of the elderly with hip fractures. In a recent report, surgical repair within the first 2 days of hospitalization and more than five sessions per week of high frequency physical and occupation therapy were associated with better health outcome (Fig. 11-1). The goal and treatment of fractures is to stabilize the fracture to allow for early mobilization. This in turn

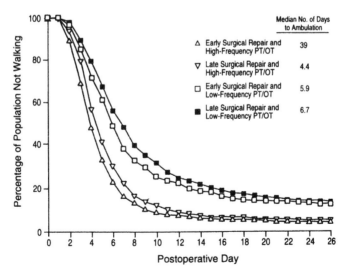

Fig. 11-1. Probability of ambulation according to timing of surgical repair and physical and occupational therapy (PT/OT). (From Arch Intern Med 157:513–520, 1997. Copyright 1997, American Medical Association.)

minimizes associated joint contractures and loss of range of motion, as well as surrounding muscle atrophy. With osteoporotic fractures, it is difficult to obtain rigid fixation by use of orthopedic hardware. Plates and screws may have suboptimal holding power. In addition, stress risers that are caused by screw holes or the end of a plate or rod may lead to further fracture. Fracture callus in osteoporosis is less abundant and less dense and less well organized. In addition, immobilization required for fracture management further accelerates local disuse osteoporosis.

Because of the difficulty with plates and screws, intermedullary rods are often preferred. They provide a mechanical advantage over plates and screws as they are positioned close to the mechanical axis of the long bone and are less prone to fatigue fracture. Rods are load sharing devices, which align the fracture fragments while at the same time permit load transmission across the fracture fragments. This helps to accelerate bone healing and promote callus formation.

As noted above, plates are dependent on the bone holding power of the screws. In osteoporosis, this is significantly compromised. Polymethylmethacrylate (PMMA) may be used to enhance initial screw fixation in osteoporotic bone. Fracture must be initially reduced and then cement can be placed in the fracture site and screws placed in the cement once it hardens. This cement can be drilled and tapped much like cortical bone. In addition, the surgeon can opt to use bolts and nuts instead of screws, but this requires a bigger dissection. With a bigger dissection comes subperiosteal striping, which compromises the blood supply and should be avoided if possible. Most vertebral compression fractures can be treated nonoperatively. This includes activity modification, pain medication, and bracing occasionally. Despite optimal nonoperative management, some spinal compression fractures do not heal and are disabling. Injection with polymethylmethacrylate under fluoroscopic control can lead to dramatic relief of pain.

Osteoporosis in Spinal Surgery

Osteoporosis presents unique problems for the spine surgeon. Correction of deformity of the spine often requires the use of hardware. Several studies have correlated instrumentation failure with decreasing bone density. This is most commonly encountered acutely in the operating room when the surgeon notes difficulty in purchase of a screw. The ability to obtain reasonable fixation in the osteoporotic patient is technique related. Low insertional torque correlates with poor purchase and also correlates with low bone mineral density. Purchase can be improved by injecting methylmethacrylate into a pedicle into which a screw has poor fixation. This has been shown to increase pull out strength by approximately 2-fold. Another way to augment the vertebral body has been recently described injecting carbonated apatite cancellous bone cement. This has also been show to increase pull out strength. Screw length may also be increased to engage the anterior cortex of the vertebrae and may be especially important in the sacrum where the anterior posterior diameter of S1 is smaller than the other vertebrae. This however carries with it some risks of vascular complication especially in the lumbar spine. Finally, increasing the screw diameter has also been shown to enhance screw fixation. Other technical factors or additional hardware such as nonparallel placement of the pedicle screws and addition of a laminar hook may help to reinforce the construct. Similarly, the addition of a sub-laminar wire may also augment a screw, which has poor purchase. The sur-geon may in some cases be faced with a situation where despite a variety of techniques it is not possible to obtain satisfactory fixation of a given mo-tion segment. At that point, the surgeon has two choices. One could perform an *in situ* fusion followed by postoperative bed rest and/or an orthosis. Al-ternatively, the instrumentation could be extended to achieve fixation in an-other level. Because of the complications associated with spinal instrumen-tation and severe osteoporosis, some surgeons feel that this is a relative contraindication to this type of surgery.

Localized Osteoporosis

Like systemic osteoporosis, when localized osteoporosis occurs, it occurs more rapidly in trabecular bone than in cortical bone. For example, with an immobilized limb, the mass of cortical bone changes little for several months. In contrast, measurable trabecular bone loss can occur in 1 week's time. There are several situation in which either pathologic condition and/or sur-gical intervention can result in localized osteoporosis.

The first and most common of these is fracture. Following fracture, muscle function in the region of the fracture markedly decreases which in turn de-creases the normal stresses seen by the bone. With reduced stress, bone atrophies. Again, trabecular bone loss occurs first and at a faster pace than cortical bone loss. With fracture healing and return to normal function, nor-mal bone loading also returns. This results in restoration of normal bone density with time in most cases. In addition, it will result in remodeling of the fracture callus so that only the callus that is loaded remains.

The use of internal fixation devices such as plates and screws can per-manently lead to localized osteoporosis. As plates can be permanent load-sharing devices, the total load normally taken by the bone is thus decreased and divided in some fashion between bone and implant. The fractured bone is therefore permanently stress shielded and atrophy and osteoporosis of the healing bone can result. In general, the use of intramedullary nail fixation is less load sharing and therefore results in less disuse osteoporosis. The gen-eral principle involved is that the greater the load sharing by the fixation de-vice, the more atrophy there will be in the bone at the site of the device. When one removes the screws and plates, it is important to remember that the screw holes are stress risers especially in bone which is more osteo-porotic than the surrounding bone. These stress risers put the patient at risk for refracture.

Birthdate: 02/05/50   Age: 41
Physician: AVIOLI

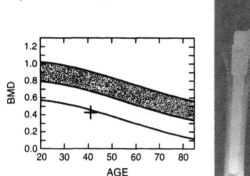

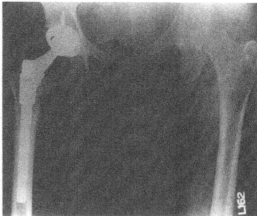

Fig. 11-2. Dual photon absorptiometry (DEXA) quantitating the left femoral neck in a 41-year-old individual with a right femoral neck prosthesis. Note that the bone mass density (BMD) of the left femoral neck (+) is less than 2 standard deviations below the mean value. (Courtesy of Louis Avioli.)

Localized osteoporosis also results following total hip or total knee arthroplasty. The bone loss may occur not only on the side of surgery but also on the contralateral limb as a result of skeletal immobilization (Fig. 11-2). Similar to fracture fixation devices, these are load sharing devices where load prior to surgery was totally taken by the bone is now shared between implant and bone. In the normal hip joint a load is transmitted proximally to distally through the femoral head and femoral neck to the cortical bone of the proximal femur. Following insertion of a femoral component in total hip arthroplasty, load transmission to the proximal femur is altered. As a result of this load sharing, the mechanical forces in the proximal femur are reduced resulting in adaptive bone remodeling which as detailed earlier leads to a decrease in bone mineral density of the proximal femur. This is evident on clinical X rays where one can compare preoperative and postoperative X rays and see a decrease in cortical thickness and density. This phenomenon has been widely referred to as stress shielding.

Localized osteoporosis can also be associated with specific diseases. The most common of those that present to the orthopedic surgeon is inflammatory arthritis such as rheumatoid arthritis. One of the first radiographic signs of rheumatoid arthritis is periarticular osteoporosis near the inflamed joint. The first radiographic abnormality noted in an infected joint may also be localized osteoporosis. The etiology of osteoporosis in these pathologic conditions is likely to be a combination of the inflammatory events which occur in the region of the disease resulting in the secretion of a variety of bone resorbing factors including prostaglandin E_2, interleukin-1, and tumor necrosis factor, as well as the mechanical events which occur as a result of pain limiting function and therefore decreasing loads to the surrounding bone.

Another pathologic entity associated with localized osteoporosis is reflux sympathetic dystrophy (RSD). This most commonly occurs as a response to a traumatic injury although the injury can be trivial in some cases. Clinical features of RSD include prolonged severe pain associated with swelling. Osteoporosis is usually limited to the painful region and is associated with vasomotor instability. Initially, clinical radiographs will often demonstrate patchy osteoporosis, which over time evolve to a more generalized localized osteoporosis. By 6 to 9 months following the initiating event, there is frequently notable cortical thinning. When the condition improves, osteoporosis also improves. It is presumed that the osteoporosis is a result of the vasomotor instability and not the cause of the condition.

Transient osteoporosis of the hip is another disease process that results in localized osteoporosis. This is a relatively rare condition most commonly occurring in pregnant women in the third trimester. The course is benign and full recovery occurs, however, it may take several months. During that time course, the patients can have severe pain and limitation of motion of the hip and require supports to walk. Radiographic analysis demonstrates marked osteopenia of the involved hip. Radionucleotide scans using technetium diphosphate show increased uptake. From the orthopedic surgeon's standpoint, it is important to distinguish transient osteoporosis of the hip from the osteonecrosis. Whereas osteonecrosis is limited to the femoral head, transient osteoporosis of the hip can involve both the head and neck of the femur. Magnetic resonance imaging can often help to distinguish between the two conditions. In addition, the degree of focal osteopenia seen with transient osteoporosis of the hip is much more significant than that seen with osteonecrosis. Again, from the surgeon's standpoint it is important to make this distinction to avoid operating on patients with transient osteoporosis.

SUGGESTED READING

Bacon WE, Maggi S, Looker A, Harris T, Nair CR, Giaconi J, Honkanen R, Ho SC, Peffers KA, Torring O, Gass R, Bonzalez N: International comparison of hip fracture rates in 1988–89. Osteoporosis Int 6:69–75, 1996.

Bagur A, Mautalen C, Rubin Z: Epidemiology of hip fractures in an urban population of central Argentina. Osteoporosis Int 4:332–335, 1994.

Barber J, Mills H, Horne G, Purdie G, Devane P: The incidence of hip fractures in Maori and non-Maori in New Zealand. N Z Med J 108:367–368, 1995.

Coe JD, Warden KE, Herzig MA, McAfee PC: Influence of bone marrow density on the fixation of thoracollumbar implants: A comparative study of transpedicular screws, laminar hooks, and spinous process wires. Spine 15:902–907, 1990.

Cooper C, Atkinson E, O'Fallon W, Melton L: Incidence of clinically diagnosed vertebral fractures: A population base study in Rochester, Minnesota, 1985–1989. J Bone Miner Res 7(2):221–227, 1992.

Dias JJ: An analysis of the nature of injury in fractures of the neck of the femur. Ageing 16:373–377, 1987.

Greenspan SL, Myers ER, Maitland LA, Resnick NM, Hayes WC: Fall severity and bone marrow density as risk factors for hip fracture in ambulatory elderly. JAMA 217:128–133, 1994.

Guidelines for preclinical evaluation and clinical trials in osteoporosis. WHO Technical Reports, WHO Geneva, Switzerland, pp 27–28, 1998.

Gullberg B, Duppe H, Nilsson BE, Redlund-Johnell I, Sernbo I, Obrant KJ, Johnell O: Incidence of hip fractures in Malmo, Sweden (1950–1991). Bone 14:S23–S29, 1993.

Hayes W, Myers E, Morris JN, Yett HS, Lipsitz LA: Impact near the hip dominates fracture risk in elderly nursing home residence who fall. Calcif Tissue Int 52:192–198, 1993.

Hoenig H, Rubenstein LV, Sloane R, Horner R, Kahan K: What is the role of timing in the surgical and rehabilitative care of community-dwelling older persons with acute hip fracture? Arch Intern Med 157:513–520, 1997.

Hughes SS, Furia JP, Smith P, Pellegrini VD Jr: Atrophy of the proximal part of the femur after total hip arthroplasty without cement. A quantitative comparison of cobalt-chromium and titanium femoral stems with use of dual x-ray absorptiometry. J Bone Joint Surg 77A:231–239, 1995.

Jacobsen SJ, Goldberg J, Miles TP, Brady JA, Stiers W, Rimm AA: Regional variation in the incidence of hip fractures: U.S. white women age 65 years and older. JAMA 264:500–502, 1990.

Jacobsen SJ, Sargent DJ, Atkinson EJ, O'Fallon WM, Melton LJ: Population-based study of the contribution of weather to hip fracture seasonality. Am J Epidemiol 141:79–83, 1995.

Kiratli BJ, Heiner JP, McBeath AA, Wilson MA: Determination of bone mineral density by dual x-ray absorptiometry in patients with uncemented total hip arthroplasty. J Orthop Res 10:836–844, 1992.

Kroger H, Venesmaa P, Jurvelin J, Miettinen H, Suomalainen O, Alhava E: Bone density at the proximal femur after total hip arthroplasty. Clin Ortho Related Res 352:66–74, 1998.

Laaritzen JB, Petersen WM, Lund B: Effect of external hip protectors on hip fracture. Lancet 341:11–13, 1993.

Maloney WJ, Sychterz C, Bragdon C, McGovern T, Jasty M, Engh CA, Harris WH: Skeletal response to well fixed femoral components inserted with and without cement. Clin Orthop 333:15–26, 1996.

Marchetti ME, Steinberg GG, Greene JM, Jenis LG, Baran DT: A prospective study of proximal femur bone mass following cemented and uncemented hip arthroplasty. J Bone Miner Res 11:1033–1039, 1996.

Melton LJ: How many people have osteoporosis now? J Bone Miner Res 10:175–177, 1995.

Melton LJ III, Atkinson EJ, Madhok R: Downturn in hip fracture incidence. Public Health Rep 111:146–150, 1996.

Michelson J, Myers A, Jinnah R, Cox Q, VanNatta M: Epidemiology of hip fractures among the elderly: Risk factors for fracture type. Clin Orthop 311:129–135, 1995.

Nevitt MC, Cummings SR: Type of fall and risk of hip and wrist fractures: The study of osteoporotic factors. J Am Geriatric Soc 41:1226–1234, 1993.

Nilsson BE, Obrant KJ: Secular tendencies of the incidence of fracture of the upper end of the femur. Acta Orthop Scand 49:389–391, 1978.

Ray WA, Griffin MR, Downey W: Benzodiazepines of long and short elimination half-life and the risk of hip fracture. JAMA 262:3303–3307, 1989.

Rogmark C, Sernbo I, Johnell O, Nilsson JA: Incidence of hip fractures in Malmo, Sweden, 1992–1995. Acta Orthop Scand 70:19–22, 1999.

Schurman DJ, Maloney WJ, Smith RL: Localized osteoporosis. In Marcus R, Feldman D, Kelsey J (eds): Osteoporosis. San Diego: Academic Press, 1996, pp 991–1008.

Scott DF, Jaffe WL: Host–bone response to porous-coated cobalt-chrome and hydroxyapatite-coated titanium femoral components in hip arthroplasty. Dual-energy x-ray absorptiometry analysis of paired bilateral cases at 5 to 7 years. J Arthroplasty 11:429–437, 1996.

12 Glucocorticoid-Related Osteoporosis

Robert Marcus

INTRODUCTION

The relationship of chronic glucocorticoid (GC) use to bone loss and frequent, occasionally devastating fractures has been recognized for almost 50 years. Few skeletal disorders have proved so vexing to treat as GC osteoporosis, but recent years have witnessed important progress in understanding this condition, its pathogenesis and prevention, and have even seen partial reversal of established disease. This chapter reviews current understanding of the causes of GC osteoporosis as well as means to prevent and treat it. Published literature in this field is vast, encompassing many animal models, both *in vitro* and *in vivo*. Unfortunately, many interesting results appear to be highly specific for a particular model. Therefore, to assure relevance to human disease, this chapter emphasizes experience in humans.

In children, chronic exposure to GCs interferes with skeletal growth and maturation. GC-induced deficits in childhood bone mass largely reflect failure of normal skeletal acquisition occasionally compounded by bone loss. In contrast, GC-induced skeletal deficits in adults exclusively reflect bone loss, due largely, but not entirely, to a disruption of the normal relationship between the resorption and formation phases of bone remodeling. The focus of this chapter will be the effects of GC in adult humans.

When adults are administered high doses of GCs for more than several days, rapid bone loss ensues. Indeed, deficits in bone mineral density (BMD) may be reliably measured within a few months of starting therapy. Bone loss in the axial (central) skeleton exceeds that in appendicular (peripheral) bone, reflecting the greater investment of trabecular bone in axial regions. Two factors explain this observation. Bone remodeling occurs only on bone surfaces, and the surface to volume ratio is greater in trabecular than in cortical bone. The cells (and their precursors) that participate in bone remodeling arise from stem cells located in red bone marrow, which in adults resides exclusively in the axial skeleton. The magnitude of axial bone loss typically approaches 40% of initial values, whereas peripheral bone loss is more likely to be about 20%.

The consequence of steroid-induced bone loss is bone fragility and an increased risk for low-trauma fractures. In the axial skeleton this translates into a particularly high incidence of vertebral compression fractures. However, as the entire skeleton of affected individuals is placed in jeopardy, fractures are more common at virtually all sites. Skeletal fragility is not the only factor contributing to fracture risk in steroid-treated patients, since steroids (and the illnesses for which they are given) are also associated with muscle weakness, which may be profound, and which itself creates instability and increases the risk for falling.

Much effort has gone into defining the patient, steroid dosage, and treatment characteristics most likely to be associated with bone loss. Many attempts to address these issues are confounded by including patients with highly variable steroid consumption patterns who suffer a wide variety of medical conditions, some of which independently contribute to poor bone health. However, some general statements seem reasonable:

1. GC-induced bone loss generally follows sustained administration of systemic doses of steroid greater than 5 mg/day of prednisone or its equivalent.

2. Skeletal consequences of steroid administration may depend on the condition that is being treated. Patients given a week-long course of high-dose prednisone to treat poison oak are not generally at risk, but frail elders with rheumatic conditions may be placed in considerable jeopardy by even low-dose steroids.

3. Used according to the manufacturer's recommendations, most steroid inhalers available in the United States pose little concern, as systemic absorption of glucocorticoids is insubstantial. However, excessive use of standard preparations may achieve systemic concentrations adequate to suppress the hypothalamic–pituitary axis and would predictably lead to loss of bone. Caution must certainly be exercised with regard to the use of recently introduced superpotent steroid products in some countries.

4. Patients treated with maintenance doses of hydrocortisone, for example, 20 mg/day, for adrenocortical insufficiency do not generally have an increased skeletal risk. However, based on accurate measurements of steroid production rates in normal humans, maintenance doses of hydrocortisone are now estimated to be lower (i.e., 15 mg/day) than have traditionally been recommended (~30 mg/day). Thus, patients who continue to be treated according to older recommendations may be at risk for excessive bone loss.

PATHOPHYSIOLOGY OF GLUCOCORTICOID OSTEOPOROSIS

Glucocorticoids affect human mineral metabolism through functional alterations in the kidney, intestine, and skeleton. Least appreciated, but occurring within a few days of initiating therapy, is a direct inhibition of renal tubular calcium reabsorption, leading to hypercalciuria. Calciuria is magnified by excessive dietary sodium, and is attenuated by coadministration of thiazide class diuretics.

Intestinal Calcium Absorption

Given at high dose for several weeks, GCs directly inhibit intestinal calcium absorption, leading to lower plasma ionized calcium activity. This is thought to stimulate compensatory hypersecretion of parathyroid hormone (PTH), which restores ionized calcium activity by increasing the efficiency of renal calcium reabsorption and by increasing the delivery of calcium from bone to the circulation through activating bone turnover. Thus, the dominant model for conceptualizing steroid-induced changes in bone homeostasis involves an increase in activity of the parathyroid axis. The operative term in this model is "activity," because it has been very difficult to show with consistency that plasma concentrations of PTH are actually elevated in steroid-treated patients. Evidence has been presented that expression of PTH action in bone and kidney may be enhanced in the presence of GC, so the described model does not require increased PTH concentrations for plausibility.

It was postulated initially that the intestinal effects of corticosteroids reflected alterations in vitamin D metabolism. However, clear-cut effects of GCs on the production, clearance, and circulating concentrations of vitamin D metabolites have not been consistently demonstrable, and it appears that the intestinal actions of GC are independent of the vitamin D system. Administration of the hormonal form of vitamin D, 1,25-dihydroxyvitamin D (calcitriol), increases, but does not normalize, fractional intestinal absorption of calcium. Despite many studies with isolated intestinal cellular and tissue preparations, the exact mechanisms by which GCs impair gut calcium absorption remain imprecisely understood. Nonetheless, when intestinal calcium absorption has been studied in patients taking high doses of GCs, low values have been observed.

Bone Remodeling

To understand the interaction of steroids with the skeleton requires a brief consideration of bone remodeling, the lifelong process of bone destruction and renewal. In adults, remodeling is fundamentally inefficient, that is to say, bone that was removed through osteoclastic resorption is not completely restored by osteoblastic bone formation. This inefficiency guarantees that any disturbance that increases overall remodeling activity will be accompanied by an increased rate of bone loss, whereas interventions aimed at slowing remodeling will attenuate it.

Glucocorticoids interact with the skeleton at multiple sites. In mice, they directly promote osteoclastic bone resorption, an effect that may not occur in primates and humans. Steroids have been consistently shown to be potent inhibitors of osteoblastic maturation and activity. In addition, recent information on the developmental program of multipotent stem cells residing in bone marrow stroma indicates that GCs shift cell maturation away from an osteoblastic lineage toward development of other cell lines, particularly adipocytes. Finally, it appears that glucocorticoids promote osteoblast cell death by apoptosis.

In a recent clinical study, prednisolone, 50 mg/day, was administered to healthy men for several months to diminish antispermatazoal antibodies. Treatment was associated with bone loss and with reduced concentrations of bone formation markers, but with no evidence for a rise in either circulating PTH or in the excretion of bone resorption markers. Thus, when the effects of steroids in humans were studied outside of the confounding influences imposed by concurrent disease or inactivity, the major skeletal effect of GCs was an inhibition of bone formation.

One additional and frequently overlooked site of steroid action is the hypothalamic–pituitary axis. High-dose corticosteroids suppress gonadotropin secretion and create a hypogonadal state in both men and women. Thus, a component of the bone loss in some steroid-treated patients is likely to be related to loss of gonadal function.

SKELETAL EVALUATION OF GLUCOCORTICOID-TREATED PATIENTS

The initial skeletal evaluation of steroid-treated patients resembles that of any patient, albeit with additional focus on the disease for which steroids are being prescribed as well as on the steroid regimen itself. The initial history should include factors known to influence peak bone mass as well as those that promote adult bone loss. Such factors include lifelong patterns of diet and physical activity; serious illness; pubertal development; menstrual history, including inquiry about sustained interruptions of postmenarcheal menstrual patterns; history of immobilization and previous fractures; use of medications that influence bone (anticonvulsant drugs, thyroid hormone, fat soluble vitamins, contraceptive medications, etc.); and family history.

With respect to GC exposure, information regarding preparations, dosage, routes of administration, and duration of use is key. In addition, it should be noted whether and how many attempts have been made to reduce steroid dosage and whether such an attempt might be reasonably made again.

Physical examination should encompass the organ systems that are affected by GCs. This includes a search for skin fragility, striae, bruising, muscle wasting, parotid swelling, and cataract formation. Accentuation of central fat depots may be obvious, with a dorsal cervical fat pad (so-called dowager's hump) and filling-in of the supraclavicular space.

Muscle strength should be assessed throughout with primary focus on proximal groups such as the quadriceps femoris complex, which may be uniquely and severely affected by GCs. Patients with steroid myopathy may be unable to rise from a chair or step onto a low stool without using their arms. For patients with rheumatologic disease, the joint flexibility, deformity, and range of motion should be noted.

Height should be measured against a wall-mounted ruler or with a stadiometer at each visit. Examination of the back should include assessment of flexibility, deformity, paraspinous muscle spasm, and point tenderness.

Laboratory Evaluation

Routine evaluation should include a complete blood count and multichannel laboratory chemistry panel. The latter should include the serum calcium concentration and alkaline phosphatase activity. A 24-h urine should be collected for calcium and creatinine concentrations, and a serum 25-hydroxyvitamin D concentration gives the best assessment of overall vitamin D nutritional state. Measurements of PTH are not generally required unless abnormalities of blood or urinary calcium are revealed. Because GCs frequently suppress the gonadal axis, it is reasonable to measure testosterone and luteinizing hormone (LH) in male patients. It should not be necessary to document circulating estrogens in women who are either amenorrheic or regularly cycling, but such assessment might be undertaken when gonadal status is not clear.

Bone Turnover Markers

Specific markers of bone resorption and formation activity have been introduced into clinical practice within the last few years. They permit noninvasive, inexpensive, and reasonably precise evaluation of the components of bone remodeling. Although they have contributed substantially to understanding of pathophysiology and to the therapeutic response of groups of participants in clinical trials, the clinical utility, if any, for bone turnover markers in managing individual patients remains uncertain. Should a physician wish to document rapid or suppressed turnover in a given patient, the urinary concentration of highly specific breakdown products of type I collagen provides a reasonably accurate estimate of bone resorption activity. Available tests include free cross-linked collagen fragments (Pyrilinks-D, Metra Biosystems, Inc., Mountain View, CA) and peptide-associated cross-links (NTx, Ostex, Inc., Seattle, WA; Crosslaps, Osteometer, Inc.). Commercially available markers of bone formation include two osteoblast-specific proteins, bone alkaline phosphatase and osteocalcin. Osteocalcin is not a useful marker to assess GC-treated patients, because production of this protein is uniquely and specifically inhibited by GCs.

Bone Mass Measurement

It is recommended to assess bone mass in all steroid treated patients except perhaps those who are so seriously afflicted by fractures and deformity that valid measurements may not be obtained and in whom clinical decisions would be compelling and straightforward even without this evaluation. It is of particular importance to obtain a bone mass measurement on patients who are just beginning or about to begin steroid treatment, since this will identify individuals with very low bone mass even before steroid exposure in whom aggressive preventive treatment would be imperative.

A discussion of various modalities for bone density measurement exceeds the scope of this chapter. Suffice it to say that when dual energy X-ray absorptiometry (DXA) is available, a combined assessment of spine, hip, and forearm bone density (BMD) by this technique is rapid, accurate, and reasonably precise, with minimal exposure to ionizing radiation. BMD determinations give valuable prognostic information and also improve follow-up of patients over time. Because of the rapidity and severity of bone loss shortly after initiating GCs, follow-up measurements can be made as early as 6 months following baseline measurements in patients whose exposure to steroids is recent. This interval will be longer for patients who have been chronically exposed to GCs because their lower rate of bone loss may require an interval of 1–2 years before valid sequential information can be expected.

Radiographs

Routine skeletal surveys of patients who have not sustained a fracture are not indicated. However, when a patient has noted loss of height or has experienced symptoms compatible with vertebral compression, lateral radiographs of the thoracic and lumbar spine are appropriate. Compression fractures may not be obvious, but a 20% diminution of anterior, middle, or posterior vertebral height compared to the other two measurements is considered to be a reasonably conservative indication of a compression fracture.

PREVENTION OF STEROID-INDUCED OSTEOPOROSIS

Modification of Steroid Dose and Spectrum

Given the notoriously poor response of glucocorticoid osteoporosis to available therapies, prevention remains the approach most likely to give a

**TABLE 12-1. Approach to Skeletal Protection
of Glucocorticoid-Treated Patients**

Minimize steroid exposure
  Taper dose
  Switch to inhaled or topical steroid
Hormone replacement therapy as needed
Supplemental calcium, vitamin D
  Calcium intake of 1500 mg/day
  Maintenance of 25-hydroxyvitamin D > 20 ng/ml
  Sodium restriction and thiazide for hypercalciuria
Exercise as tolerated
  Weight-bearing for skeletal loading
  Strength training to maintain muscle function
BMD assessment (spine and hip) every 6 months for first 2 years, annually thereafter
Antiresorptive medication
  Calcitriol for marginal vitamin D/calcium status
  Bisphosphonates
  Calcitonin
Promising agents under investigation
  Parathyroid hormone
  Calcitriol analogs

Adapted from Lukert B: Glucocorticoid-induced osteoporosis. In Marcus R, Feldman D, Kelsey J, eds: Osteoporosis. San Diego: Academic Press, 1996, pp 801–820.

favorable outcome (Table 12-1). Perhaps the most important aspect of a sound preventive strategy is to limit exposure to corticosteroids and to find alternative treatments if at all possible. If a patient requires a high steroid dose to enter remission for a particular disorder, the physician should always be sensitive to opportunities for initiating a dose reduction or switching to nonsystemic forms of steroids, such as inhaled or topical steroids. Unfortunately, the use of alternate-day steroids, which is known to protect growth in steroid-treated children, appears not to offer skeletal protection to steroid-treated adults.

The possibility that a bone-sparing glucocorticoid might be developed has been a matter of discussion for many years. Such a drug ideally would possess full anti-inflammatory actions without jeopardizing the skeleton. To date, no such agent has been approved in the United States. Deflazacort, a synthetic oxazoline derivative of prednisolone, is reported to be less harmful to cancellous bone than other corticosteroids of equal anti-inflammatory potency. *In vitro,* deflazacort and cortisol produce similar inhibition of osteoblast proliferation and collagen synthesis, whereas cortisol appears to be more effective an inhibitor of insulin-like growth factor (IGF-I) production. In a clinical trial comparing deflazacort to prednisone, both steroids resulted in trabecular bone loss, but that induced by prednisone exceeded that associated with deflazacort. However, it remains possible that this apparent "protective" effect could simply represent lower total effective glucocorticoid exposure. Recent development of selective estrogen-receptor modulators (SERMs), such as raloxifene, lends optimism that an agent can be engineered that selectively activates glucocorticoid receptors in a tissue-specific manner as well.

In patients who require immunosuppression following organ transplantation, widespread use of cyclosporine and tacrolimus has permitted substantial reductions in GC use. However, these newer drugs have been clearly shown to increase bone turnover and promote bone loss, so the net effect on bone status may be just as worrisome as GC.

Calcium and Vitamin D Support

The rationale for providing supplemental calcium and vitamin D to steroid treated patients is that this intervention will raise the ionized calcium activity in plasma, suppress PTH secretion, and thereby reduce the rate of bone remodeling. By doing so, the number of remodeling units in action at any given time is minimized and accumulation of BMD deficits is reduced. So long as the patient continues to take GCs, however, this approach will not reverse the inhibition of osteoblast recruitment, action, or survival. In general, patients should receive 1500 mg/day of supplemental calcium. Various schedules of vitamin D support have been used, ranging from 400 international units (IU)/day to 50,000 IU three times/week.

Physical Activity

The skeleton responds to immobilization by bone loss, so inactivity must be avoided in steroid treated patients when at all possible. Some conditions such as polymyalgia rheumatica respond exuberantly to steroid therapy, giving patients a rapid and complete recovery of function. These patients may have little difficulty maintaining a vigorous schedule of weight-bearing activities during treatment. Patients with other conditions may not regain full mobility and may have residual functional disabilities. It is particularly important for those patients to receive physical therapy or other appropriate assistance for maintaining and restoring functional capacity.

Hormone Replacement Therapy

The ability of glucocorticoids to inhibit the hypothalamic–pituitary–gonadal axis has been referred to above. In some rheumatologic conditions, such as systemic lupus erythematosus, estrogens have been traditionally avoided. When contraindications to estrogen do not exist, replacement therapy will protect bone mass.

SPECIFIC PHARMACOLOGIC THERAPY OF STEROID-INDUCED OSTEOPOROSIS

Drug therapy for skeletal disorders is conventionally divided into agents that act to inhibit resorption and those that stimulate bone formation. Recent years have witnessed a series of controlled clinical trials of calcium and vitamin D, vitamin D analogs, the peptide hormone calcitonin, and bisphosphonates in steroid-treated patients. Calcium, vitamin D, and the vitamin D analogs increase net intestinal calcium absorption, thereby suppressing the parathyroid axis. As this effect leads to a reduction in bone resorption, such therapy is, strictly speaking, antiresorptive. All of the other listed agents are directly antiresorptive; that is, they suppress the proliferation and maturation of osteoclast precursors and/or inhibit the actions of mature osteoclasts.

Calcitriol and Calcitonin

In a large clinical trial, patients starting long-term GC were given 1000 mg supplemental calcium and either the potent vitamin D metabolite, $1,25\text{-}(OH)_2$ vitamin D (calcitriol) (up to 1 μg/day) plus salmon calcitonin (400 units/day by nasal spray), calcitriol alone, or placebo for 1 year. Preservation of lumbar spine BMD was observed in subjects who received calcitriol, either alone or with calcitonin, compared with those who received placebo or calcium alone, but no benefit was observed at the femoral neck.

Several points can be made from this study. First, even though bone loss was observed in subjects treated only with calcium, it was of a lower magnitude than would otherwise have been predicted. Thus, calcium supplementation appeared to be a useful adjunctive treatment. Second, patients treated with calcitriol experienced significantly less bone loss from the spine than did those who did not receive this agent. It is not certain whether the addition of calcitonin to the calcitriol regimen conferred additional benefit. These results confirm a unique predilection of GC bone loss for the spine, and support the clinical utility of calcitriol in protection against such loss. In this study, calcitonin emerged as only of marginal value. However, in patients who do not tolerate other, more potent medications, calcitonin may safely be used. In addition, a number of investigators have described a potential analgesic effect of this agent when given to patients with painful compression fractures. One area of concern regarding calcitriol is its tendency in several trials to produce hypercalciuria and hypercalcemia. Consequently, if a physician decides to use this agent, routine frequent monitoring of urine and blood calcium concentrations is mandatory.

Bisphosphonates

In light of the fact that the primary skeletal abnormality induced by GC is an inhibition of bone formation, the potential benefits of potent antiresorptive agents are not immediately obvious. Nonetheless, well-conducted trials have shown unequivocal benefit in terms of conserving and even increasing bone density. In one recent study, cyclic etidronate (Didronel) (400 mg/day for 14 days every 3 months) was given to patients recently started on high-dose GC for multiple indications. While patients treated with placebo lost about 3% of BMD from spine and hip, treatment with etidronate led to increases in BMD of 0.6 and 1.5%, respectively. In addition, the active treatment group experienced significantly fewer vertebral fractures than did the placebo group.

In a study of patients who had been treated with GC for variable periods of time, 48 weeks of daily alendronate (5 or 10 mg/day) significantly increased BMD of the spine and hip compared to a control group (Saag *et al.,* 1998) (Fig. 12-1). This response was independent of the duration of steroid use prior to initiating treatment. In this study, trends in vertebral fracture incidence did not meet statistical significance, and nonvertebral fractures were equally common in active and placebo groups. However, the fact that many of the participants in this trial had been taking GC long term may have biased the study toward individuals whose skeletal fragility was so great that fracture would still be a likely occurrence even after a year of effective therapy. Once again, these results indicate that the optimum time to initiate skeletal protection against GC is early in the course of steroid treatment. In a 2-year follow-up presentation at an international scientific meeting, the same authors reported that alendronate resulted in a 90% reduction in vertebral fracture, although an apparent reduction in nonvertebral fractures remained nonsignificant.

One issue concerning bisphosphonates that is a persistent concern is the occurrence of adverse events, particularly esophageal irritation. In both of these bisphosphonate trials, the medications were well tolerated. Despite simultaneous administration of corticosteroids and other anti-inflammatory drugs, no increase in esophageal symptoms or ulceration was encountered in the active treatment groups for either study. However, some patients are unable to tolerate oral bisphosphonates. In such instances, pamidronate (Aredia) can be administered as an intravenous infusion (60 mg i.v. in isotonic saline, given over 4 h). This potent bisphosphonate is similar to alendronate in its antiresorptive actions and its parenteral administration completely obviates the issue of gastrointestinal toxicity.

Promoters of Bone Formation

It appears sensible that an agent that directly promotes osteoblast function would be ideal for counteracting the effects of GC. Several compounds

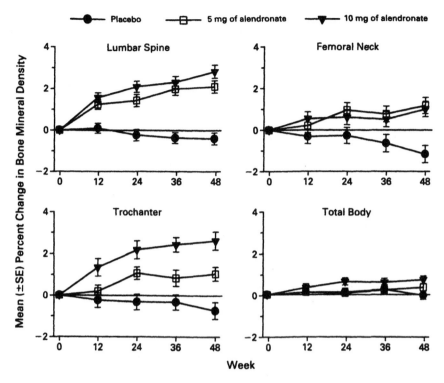

Fig. 12-1. Effects of alendronate on bone mineral density in all patients receiving an average daily dose of at least 7.5 mg of prednisone (or its equivalent). (Reproduced from Saag KG, Emkey R, Schnitzer TJ, Brown JP, Hawkins F, *et al.*: Alendronate for the prevention and treatment of glucocorticoid-induced osteoporosis. N Engl J Med 339: 292–299, 1998. Copyright © 1998 Massachusetts Medical Society. All rights reserved.)

have generated interest. The strongest evidence for a true bone anabolic effect has emerged for parathyroid hormone (PTH) and its active synthetic analogs. That PTH might stimulate osteoblasts to increase bone mass may seem counterintuitive, given the knowledge that patients with severe primary hyperparathyroidism may have profound bone disease. However, that pathological state is associated with continuously high circulating concentrations of PTH. When the hormone is given as single daily injections, a pulsatile pattern of peak and trough concentrations is achieved, and this has been associated with increased bone mass. Indeed, administration of PTH to osteoporotic women has achieved substantial gains in BMD, particularly at the lumbar spine. This agent is currently undergoing large-scale clinical trials for treatment of postmenopausal osteoporosis.

In a very recent study, hPTH(1–34), an active fragment of human PTH, was given to estrogen-replaced postmenopausal women who were taking

GC, primarily for rheumatoid arthritis. Over 1 year of follow-up, lumbar spine BMD in the group receiving the PTH analog increased by 35% (measured by computed tomography, CT) and by 11% (using DXA). By contrast, the HRT alone group experienced changes of less than 2%. The differential response between CT and DXA reflects the fact that CT specifically measures trabecular bone, which appears to have been the primary responding tissue, whereas DXA measures both trabecular bone and the surrounding cortex. These results suggest that PTH may have great clinical utility in GC-treated patients and emphasize the need for a longer-term controlled clinical trial of this agent.

Growth hormone (GH) and insulin-like growth factor I (IGF-I) both initiate bone turnover and promote bone gain in growing animals. Since GCs inhibit IGF-I production in cultured bone cells, a plausible rationale exists for trying these agents in experimental GC-osteoporosis. However, despite some interesting results in animal models, there is currently no evidence of clinical utility for either GH or IGF-I in GC-treated humans.

Fluoride salts have been used in steroid treated patients for more than 2 decades. Despite the ability of fluoride to stimulate even enormous increases in lumbar spine BMD, clinical experience worldwide has been mixed at best, with major concerns about drug safety. A delayed release form of sodium fluoride tested in postmenopausal osteoporotic women has been reported to lower the incidence of vertebral fracture. This preparation has been under consideration by the U.S. FDA for more than 2 years, but contradictory experience with fluoride in large European trials has led the regulatory agency to be very cautious. Whether slow-release fluoride will ultimately receive FDA approval is currently unknown. If that were to happen, its utility in managing GC treated patients would be an important focus of additional study.

SUGGESTED READING

Adachi JD, Bensen WG, Brown J, Hanley D, Hodsman A, Josse R, Kendler DL, Lentle B, Olszynski W, Ste-Marie L-G, Tenenhouse A, Chines AA: Intermittent etidronate therapy to prevent corticosteroid-induced osteoporosis. N Engl J Med 337:382–387, 1997.

Canalis E, Avioli L: Effects of deflazacort on aspects of bone formation in cultures of intact calvariae and osteoblast-enriched cells. J Bone Miner Res 7:1085–1092, 1992.

de Groen PC, Lubbe DF, Hirsh LJ: Esophagitis associated with the use of alendronate. N Engl J Med 335:1016–1021, 1996.

Lane NE, Sanchez S, Modin GW, Genant HK, Pierini E, Arnaud CD: Parathyroid hormone treatment can reverse corticosteroid-induced osteoporosis: Results of a randomized controlled clinical trial. J Clin Invest 102:1627–1633, 1998.

Lindsay R, Nieves J, Formica C, Henneman E, Woelfert L, Shen V, Dempster D, Cosman F: Randomised controlled study of effect of parathyroid hormone on vertebral-bone mass and fracture incidence among postmenopausal women on oestrogen with osteoporosis. Lancet 350:550–555, 1997.

LoCascio V, Ballanti P, Milani S, Bertoldo F, LoCascio C, Zanolin EM, Bonucci E: A histomorphometric long-term longitudinal study of trabecular bone loss in glucocorticoid-treated patients: Prednisone versus deflazacort. Calcif Tissue Int 62:199–204, 1998.

Lukert B: Glucocorticoid-induced osteoporosis. In Marcus R, Feldman D, Kelsey J, eds: Osteoporosis. San Diego: Academic Press, 1996, pp 801–820.

Pearce G, Ryan PF, Delmas PD, Tabensky DA, Seeman E: The deleterious effects of low-dose corticosteroids on bone density in patients with polymyalgia rheumatica. Br J Rheumatol 37:292–299, 1998.

Pearce G, Tabensky DA, Delmas PD, Baker HW, Seeman E: Corticosteroid-induced bone loss in men. J Clin Endocrinol Metab 83:801–806, 1998.

Saag K, Emkey R, Cividino A, Brown J, Goemaere S, Dumortier T, Daifotis AG, Czachur M: Effects of alendronate for two years on BMD and fractures in patients receiving glucocorticoids. Bone 23:S183 (abstract 1141), 1998.

Saag KG, Emkey R, Schnitzer TJ, Brown JP, Hawkins F, Goemare S, Thamsborg G, Liberman UA, Delmas PD, Malico M-P, Czachur M, Daifotis AG: Alendronate for the prevention and treatment of glucocorticoid-induced osteoporosis. N Engl J Med 339:292–299, 1998.

Sambrook P, Birmingham J, Kelly P, Kempler S, Nguyen T, Pocock N, Eisman J: Prevention of corticosteroid osteoporosis. A comparison of calcium, calcitriol, and calcitonin. N Engl J Med 328:1747–1752, 1993.

van Staa T, Abenhaim L, Cooper C: Upper gastrointestinal adverse events and cyclical etidronate. Am J Med 103:462–467, 1997.

13 Osteoporosis and the Bone Biopsy

Steven L. Teitelbaum

INTRODUCTION

Physicians dealing with postmenopausal patients are frequently confronted with vertebral, wrist, and/or hip fractures. The monotony of this syndrome and its association with cessation of ovarian function has led many
to consider it a reflection of a single pathogenetic mechanism. There are,
however, many senescent changes apart from ovarian failure that may lead
to postmenopausal bone loss. These include diminished renal function, alterations in vitamin D metabolism, and decreased efficiency of intestinal absorption of calcium. Undoubtedly, other factors predisposing toward postmenopausal bone loss still await discovery. It is, therefore, apparent that
the genesis of postmenopausal "osteoporosis" is complex. Histologic analysis of the senescent female skeleton only underscores the degree of this
complexity.

THE BONE BIOPSY

Postmenopausal osteoporosis belongs to the family of "metabolic" bone
diseases. The commonality of these diseases is their generalized distribution
throughout the skeleton. As such, a sample of bone taken from one site reflects changes occurring in the skeleton at large. This realization has led to
the use of the random (blind) biopsy in the histologic evaluation of the osteopenic skeleton. The iliac crest is the favored site of biopsy of patients

with generalized disorders of bone. There are a number of specifically designed trocars available for this procedure, which entails a minimum of trauma and has high patient acceptability. The biopsy can be easily performed in an outpatient setting using local anesthesia. The surgical approach yields a core of bone that includes cortices and intervening trabeculae.

The major advance in the histologic evaluation of the osteoporotic skeleton, however, is the development of techniques to prepare well-preserved, nondecalcified histologic sections. In the general histology laboratory, bone is routinely decalcified prior to sectioning. Such an approach makes a distinction between mineralized and nonmineralized (osteoid) bone matrix impossible and, therefore, obviates identification of patients with abnormalities of skeletal calcification. On the other hand, a number of laboratories now have the capacity to avoid bone decalcification when preparing histologic slides. These methods involve plastic embedding and the use of a heavy-duty microtome. The microscopic sections prepared in this manner permit easy identification of both calcified bone and osteoid (Fig. 13-1, see color plate).

The nondecalcified bone biopsy was developed primarily to distinguish osteoporosis from osteomalacia. Osteoporosis is a histologic entity defined as a decreased mass of normally mineralized bone. As such, the quantity of bone matrix per unit marrow space is diminished, but the ratio of osteoid/calcified tissue is normal.

Osteomalacia is also a histologic entity, namely, osteoid accumulation resulting from a decrease in the rate of its mineralization. Osteomalacic bone must, therefore, contain an increased quantity of uncalcified matrix (Fig. 13-2). Because osteoid is radiolucent, the roentgenographic appearance

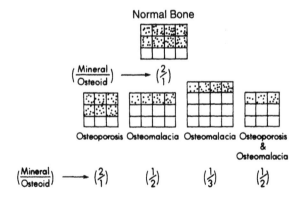

Fig. 13-2. Schematic representation of bone mass and mineral/osteoid relationships in osteoporosis and osteomalacia. Each large block represent a hypothetical bone segment. The stippled areas denote mineralized osteoid; the clear areas denote poorly mineralized or nonmineralized osteoid. The total number of small blocks in each hypothetical bone segment represents individual bone units. Note that bone mass is always decreased in osteoporosis, although the mineral/osteoid ratio is normal. Although bone mass may be normal, increased, or (when associated with osteoporosis) decreased in osteomalacia, the mineral/osteoid ratio is always decreased.

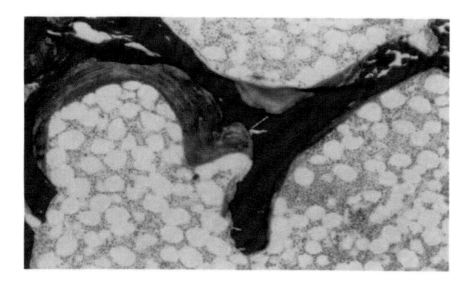

Fig. 13-1. Non-decalcified histologic section of the bone. The red material is osteoid and the blue material is mineralized bone (100 x).

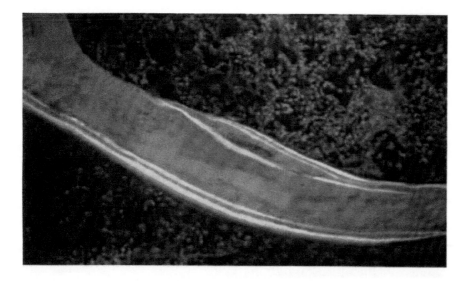

Fig. 13-4. Flourescent micrograph of bone biopsy in a patient with "high turnover" osteoporosis following administration of two, time-spaced doses of fluorescent tetracycline. The first and second doses are represented by fluorescent lines. The quantity of bone mineralized in the interdose period is reflected, and measurable by the distance between fluorescent bands and the percentage of bone surface exhibiting double labels. Active osteopenia is characterized by abundant double label formation (undecalcified, unstained fluorescent micrograph. 250 x).

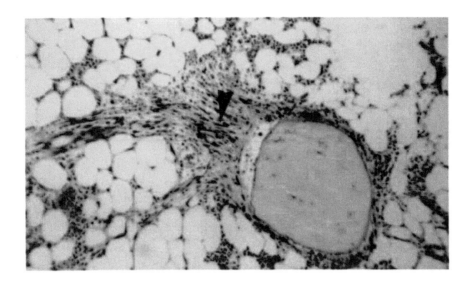

Fig. 13-7. Spindle-shaped mast cell granulomata (arrow) in the bone marrow of a patient with diffuse osteoporosis (see Fig. 13-4) subjected to a bone biopsy.

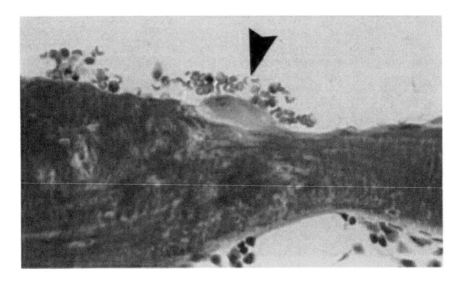

Fig. 13-8. Bone biopsy from iliac crest of patient with "high-turnover" osteoporosis. Trabecular mineralized bone is in blue; large arrow points to large osteoclast. Note increased osteoid (red) and small cells (osteoblasts) on surface opposite to osteoclast.

of osteomalacic and osteoporotic skeletons are generally identical. Even the time-honored "pseudofracture" considered the hallmark of osteomalacia (Fig. 13-3) is not invariably pathognomonic of osteomalacia. Moreover, although many moderate-to-severe cases of osteomalacia often present with aberration in biological markers of bone remodeling, patients with early osteomalacic syndromes, which can produce pain, often exhibit no distinctive biochemical abnormalities. Consequently, the radiologist and internist are usually confronted with decreased bone mass of undetermined etiology and can only make a generic diagnosis of "osteoporosis." On the other hand, the presence of excess osteoid is not, even by histologic evaluation, diagnostic of osteomalacia. Insight into this problem requires appreciation of the sequence of bone synthesis.

Bone is synthesized by the deposition of organic matrix (osteoid) and its subsequent mineralization. The duration from deposition of the molecule of osteoid, which is largely collagen, to its subsequent calcification is known as the mineralization lag time, which in humans averages 23.5 days. Osteomalacia is characterized by prolongation of the mineralization lag time.

As a result of these findings, it is obvious that osteoid accumulation may reflect one of two kinetic abnormalities, namely, (1) delayed mineralization of organic matrix (osteomalacia) or (2) enhanced rate of osteoid synthesis. Because the bone biopsy represents bone "sampling" at an isolated moment in time, it is impossible using standard, tinctorial stains, to distinguish between these two kinetic events. Fortunately, however, the skeleton is the one organ system in humans whose rate of formation may be evaluated by a single biopsy. This approach is dependent on the use of tetracyclines and their ability to chelate newly deposited bone mineral and the fluorescence of the mineral–tetracycline complex.

Bone mineral is deposited at the interface of osteoid and calcified matrix at a site known as the calcification (mineralization) front. The precise form in which the mineral first appears is enigmatic, but within a short period of time it undergoes transformation into a more "mature" phase, which comprises the majority of the adult skeleton. Following administration of tetracycline, the antibiotic binds to newly deposited (immature) bone mineral and, when examined by fluorescent microscopy, the complex appears as a yellow or orange line at the calcification front. Hence, osteoid seams that are actively undergoing mineralization exhibit a tetracycline label, while the calcification fronts of those seams that are not being mineralized fail to fluoresce. Osteomalacia is characterized by an abundance of such nonfluorescent calcification fronts.

As valuable as this determination is, it still represents an isolated moment in time and offers no information regarding the rate of mineralization. Kinetic data may be obtained, however, by using time-spaced histologic markers of mineralization.

Under these circumstances, two courses of tetracycline are given separated by a known period of time. In our practice, two 3-day courses of the antibiotic are administered separated by a 14-day interval. Such an approach results in the appearance of two parallel fluorescent bands adjacent to most

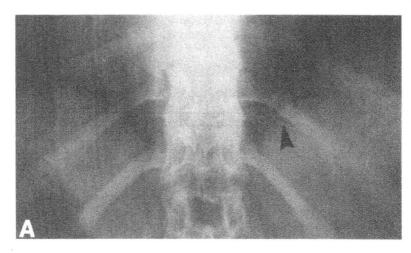

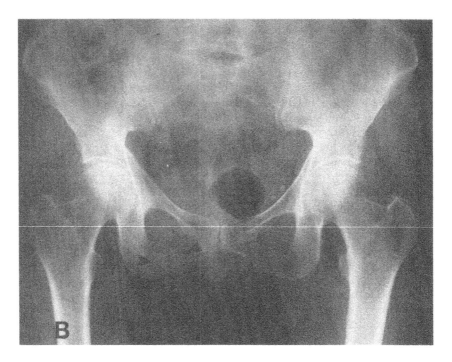

Fig. 13-3. Osteomalacia with pseudofracture and "Looser's zones" in ribs (arrow Fig. 13-3A) and pelvis (arrow Fig. 13-3B).

mineralizing osteoid seams (Fig. 13-4, see color plate). The deeper label represents the first course of antibiotic, and the more superficial one, located at the calcification front, represents the second. The mineral apposition rate, which is the rate of calcification occurring at the average point on a bone-forming surface, is calculated by determining the mean distance between parallel labels and dividing that distance by the interdose duration. If, for example, the mean distance between labels is 14 μm and the interdose duration is 14 days, it enables one to identify the kinetic abnormality leading to various states of excess osteoid (hyperosteoidosis). If the cellular rate of mineralization (bone mineral apposition rate) is diminished, excessively thick osteoid seams must reflect osteomalacia. Alternatively, if this kinetic determinant of calcification is at least normal, organic matrix synthesis is accelerated.

BONE CELL FUNCTION

Bone consists of a small number of cells in a vast organic and inorganic matrix. Despite their relatively small numbers, bone cells dictate the structure of the skeleton by its continual synthesis and degradation. For example, the anatomy of skeletal collagen reflects the rate at which it is synthesized. Normal adult bone collagen is deposited in a lamellar fashion, which when examined by polarizing microscopy appears as parallel fibers of uniform diameter. When skeletal synthesis is markedly accelerated, such as accompanies fracture repair or various states of hyperparathyroidism, collagen assumes a woven arrangement consisting of variously sized, randomly arranged fibers. The structural superiority of lamellar as compared to woven collagen underscores the fact that skeletal stability reflects both qualitative and quantitative factors.

Bone cell functions may be divided into those occurring only prior to cessation of growth and those ongoing throughout life. Growth and modeling are the processes whereby bone increases in size and is sculpted to adult proportions, respectively (Fig. 13-5). Both of these activities cease with physeal closure. Repair and remodeling, in contrast, are always extant. Repair heals fractures, and remodeling is intimately related to mineral homeostasis. Postmenopausal osteoporosis, like virtually all adult-acquired generalized skeletal diseases, is a disorder of remodeling. Hence, understanding adult osteopenia requires understanding remodeling.

The interesting aspect of remodeling, as compared to the other three cellular functions of bone, is its unique anatomic coupling of osteoclasts and osteoblasts (Fig. 13-6). Osteoclasts are the large multinucleated cells that are the principal, if not exclusive resorbers of bone, and osteoblasts are responsible for its synthesis and mineralization. Remodeling involves the activities of both cells.

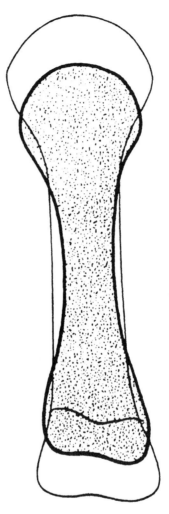

Fig. 13-5. Growth and modeling of bone. Growth refers to the increase in size of a developing (stippled) bone to its adult counterpart (open). Modeling is the sculpturing of bone or its movement through space, which must occur for maintenance of normal gross architecture. Note that modeling requires synthesis of bone on some surfaces and resorption on others. [Reproduced from Bone and Mineral Research Annual 2. In Peck, WA (ed): New York: Elsevier, 1984. With permission.]

At any time there are numerous foci of remodeling throughout the skeleton. Such a focus is initiated by the appearance of osteoclasts on a trabecular surface or within the cortex. These cells degrade a packed of bone, forming a Howship's lacuna, also known as a "resorption bay." When osteoclastic

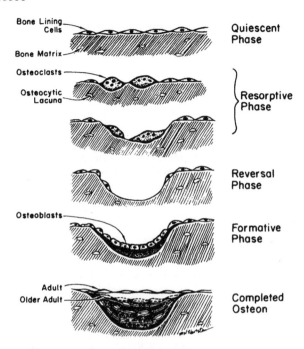

Fig. 13-6. The remodeling sequence of bone is initiated by osteoclastic resorption of indeterminate duration followed by the absence of osteoclasts or osteoblasts (the reversal phase). Subsequently, osteoblasts appear within the resorptive bay (Howship's lacuna) and synthesize matrix (the formative phase) until a new packet of bone (the osteon) is produced. In nongrowing, young adults the amounts of matrix resorbed and synthesized are in equilibrium, in older individuals, on the other hand, the amount of new bone is less than the amount removed, resulting in a net decrease in skeletal mass or osteoporosis. [Reproduced from Bone and Mineral Research Annual 2. In Peck, WA (ed): New York: Elsevier, 1984. With permission.]

activity ceases, osteoblasts appear within the cavity. The quantity of bone deposited by these cells in a Howship's lacuna need not equal that previously resorbed. In fact, the universality of bone loss with age is due to remodeling osteoblasts incompletely refilling resorption bays. Clearly, the coupling of osteoclasts and osteoblasts in remodeling is anatomic and not kinetic. Consequently, a direct relationship exists between the number of osteoclasts and osteoblasts in postmenopausal osteoporosis as well as other metabolic diseases of bone. Moreover, most perturbation that alters the number of one cell type will in a parallel fashion, influence the population of the other. It is this tethering of osteoclasts and osteoblasts which ultimately conditions the teleological approach for treating postmenopausal osteoporosis.

The development of techniques whereby osteoclasts and osteoblasts may be isolated and generated in culture has provided major insights into the

means by which these cells respectively resorb and synthesize bone. Osteoclasts are members of the monocyte/macrophage family whose resorptive
function depends on development of a microenvironment at the cell/bone
interface. This space, which is isolated from the interstices of the cell as well
as the general extracellular compartment, is acidified by a proton pump similar to that expressed by the intercalated cell of the renal tuble. Given the
difference between the pH within the resorptive microenvironment and the
extracellular space, physical intimacy must exist between the osteoclast and
bone for matrix resorption to precede. Such intimacy is mediated by the integrin $\alpha_v \beta_3$, blockade of which prevents experimental postmenopausal osteoporosis. Thus, the osteoclast proton pump and the $\alpha_v \beta_3$ integrin present
themselves as potential antiosteoporosis therapeutic targets.

THE ROLE OF BONE BIOPSY IN OSTEOPOROSIS

The nondecalcified bone biopsy has been an invaluable tool in diagnosing and following treatment of numerous metabolic disorders of bone, the
most striking example of which may be renal osteodystrophy. This family of
skeletal disorders that accompanies renal failure is now remarkably well understood and largely treatable and preventable, the latter as a result of the
availability of the nondecalcified bone biopsy. In fact, histologic examination is the most effective means of documenting aluminum-induced osteodystrophy. The bone biopsy can often prove to be diagnostic in osteoporotic
syndromes especially in patients with nonsecreting forms of multiple myeloma, and others with systemic mastocytosis (Fig. 13-7, see color plate). Patients with osteomalacia often remain misdiagnosed, since blood levels of
25-(OH)D$_3$ (which is a specific index of vitamin D sufficiency in humans)
may prove misleading in this regard.

The potential of the bone biopsy in treating the osteoporotic patient can
be utilized in order to characterize the cellular aspects of the osteoporotic
process. Postmenopausal osteoporosis is a heterogeneous disorder at the
cellular level, the latter reflecting a spectrum of kinetic changes within the
skeleton. Specifically, patients may present with either high, normal, or low
turnover bone disease. In high turnover (or active) osteoporosis, the activities of osteoclasts and osteoblasts are accelerated, while in the low turnover
(or inactive) phase of the disease, bone cell functions is generally suppressed. Normal turnover osteoporosis is characterized by diminished bone
mass accompanied by normal rates of bone formation and resorption. Histologic evidence of low turnover osteoporosis is characteristic in elderly individuals with decreased osteoblast activity and/or content (see Fig. 13-8,
see color plate). It must be realized that both high and low turnover osteoporosis are attended by a net rate of resorption (i.e., resorption minus formation) in excess of normal. On the other hand, normal turnover osteoporotic syndromes may appear in patients who achieve an insufficient peak

skeletal mass in their younger years and, therefore, become osteoporotic despite a normal net rate of bone loss.

Finally, it is important to realize that the bone biopsy cannot replace the bone mass measurement procedures described for diagnosing diminished bone mass. While other histologic features are relatively constant within the iliac crest, there is wide variation in bone mass. In this regard, we should be reminded that although a variety of osteoporotic metabolic bone disorders involve trabecular bone, approximately 20% of the skeleton is composed of trabecular bone, the remainder or 80% consisting of cortical bone. Hence, the trocar-derived bone biopsy must still be considered as an imprecise means of diagnosing generalized osteopenia. The logical approach would, therefore, include the diagnosis of osteoporosis by noninvasive techniques as detailed and, when deemed appropriate, characterization of the osteoporotic disorder by iliac crest bone biopsy procedures.

SUGGESTED READING

Chines A, Pacifici R, Avioli LV, Teitelbaum SL, Korenblat PE: Systemic mastocytosis presenting as osteoporosis: A clinical and histomorphometric study. J Clin Endocrinol Metab 72:140–144, 1991.

Darby AJ, Meunier PJ: Mean wall thickness and formation periods of trabecular bone packets in idiopathic osteoporosis. Calcif Tissue Int 33:199–204, 1981.

Fallon MD, Whyte MP, Teitelbaum SL: Systemic mastocytosis associated with generalized osteopenia. Hum Pathol 12:813–820, 1981.

Hesp R, Arlot ME, Edouard C, Bradbeer JN, Meunier PJ, Reeve J: Iliac trabecular bone formation predicts radial trabecular bone density changes in type I osteoporosis. J Bone Miner Res 6:929–935, 1991.

Johnston CC, Norton J, Khairi MRA, Kernek C, Edouard C, Arlot M, Meunier PJ: Heterogeneity of fracture syndromes in postmenopausal women. J Clin Endocrinol Metab 61:551–556, 1985.

Podenphant J, Gottredsen A, Nilas, L, Norgaard H, Braendstrup O: Iliac crest biopsy: Representativity for the amount of mineralized bone. Bone 7:427–430, 1986.

Rao SD, Matkovic V, Duncan H: Tansiliac bone biopsy. Henry Ford Hosp Med J 28(2):112–126, 1980.

Recker RR, Kimmel DB, Parfitt Am, Davies M, Keshawarx N, Hinders S: Static and tetracyline-based bone histomorphometric data from 34 normal postmenopausal females. J Bone Miner Res 3:133–144, 1988.

Teitelbaum SL: Metabolic and other nontumorous disorders of bone. In Anderson WAD, Kissane JM (eds): Pathology, 7th Ed. St. Louis: Mosby, 1977, pp 1905–1977.

Teitelbaum SL, Bullough PG: The pathophysiology of bone and joint disease. Am J Pathol 96:279–354, 1979.

Teitelbaum SL, Tondravi MM, Ross FP: Osteoclasts, macrophages, and the molecular mechanisms of bone resorption. J Leukocyte Biol 61:381–388, 1997.

Whyte MP, Bergfeld MA, Murphy WA, Avioli LV, Teitelbaum SL: Postmenopausal osteoporosis: A heterogeneous disorder as assessed by histomorphometric analysis of iliac crest bone from untreated patients. Am J Med 72:193–202, 1982.

Index

Osteoporosis, *see* Localized osteoporosis; Senile osteoporosis;
Steroid-induced osteoporosis

P

PABM, *see* Peak adult bone mass
Pamidronate, *see also* Bisphosphonates
administration routes, 127–128
bone density trials, 127–128
doses, 127
Parathyroid hormone (PTH)
bone remodeling role, 91–92
calcium effects on levels, 91–92
regulation of secretion, 30
secretion increase in aging, 28–
29, 33, 105
steroid-induced osteoporosis
prevention, 183–184
therapy effects on vertebral bone
mineral density, 154
Peak adult bone mass (PABM)
bone loss diagnosis utilization,
50–51, 54–55
importance in fracture prevention, 102
puberty onset effects in men, 27
Phytoestrogens
food content, 152
genistein effects on bone density,
153
menopausal symptom effects,
153
PICP, *see* Collagen type I propeptides
PINP, *see* Collagen type I propeptides
Precision, bone mineral density
measurements, 46, 48–49,
61–62
Preferred provider organization,
see Managed care
Prevalence, osteoporosis
age dependence, 2, 19
ethnic group rates, 2–3
trend predictions, 4, 37, 161

Progesterone
inclusion in estrogen replacement therapy, 111, 108, 111
levels following menopause, 104
PTH, *see* Parathyroid hormone
Puberty, timing and peak bone density in men, 27

Q

QCT, *see* Quantitative computed to-
mography
Quality assurance, bone mineral
density testing, 49
Quantitative computed tomography
(QCT)
central measurement principles,
47–48
Medicare fee schedule, 9
Quantitative ultrasound (QUS)
central measurement principles,
48
Medicare fee schedule, 9
QUS, *see* Quantitative ultrasound

R

RA, *see* Radiographic absorptiometry
Radiographic absorptiometry (RA),
principles, 48
Raloxifene
bone loss prevention efficacy,
113, 115
breast cancer prevention, 116
cardioprotective effects, 115–116
side effects, 116
Referral, primary care provider to
specialist, 18–19
Reflux sympathetic dystrophy
(RSD), localized osteoporosis,
170
Remodeling, *see* Bone formation;
Bone resorption
Renal osteodystrophy, bone biopsy,
194
Rheumatoid arthritis, localized osteoporosis, 169

Printed and bound by CPI Group (UK) Ltd, Croydon, CR0 4YY

03/10/2024

01040399-0003